DATE DUE

9/23/09			

Demco

DEVIANT NURSES AND IMPROPER PATIENT CARE

DEVIANT NURSES
AND IMPROPER PATIENT CARE
A Study of Failure in the Medical Profession

Ursula A. Falk
and
Gerhard Falk

The Edwin Mellen Press
Lewiston•Queenston•Lampeter

Library of Congress Cataloging-in-Publication Data

Falk, Ursula A.
  Deviant nurses and improper patient care : a study of failure in the medical profession /
by Ursula A. Falk and Gerhard Falk.
      p. cm.
  Includes bibliographical references and index.
  ISBN 13: 978-0-7734-5967-0
  ISBN 10: 0-7734-5967-7
  1. Nurses--Attitudes. 2. Nursing errors. 3. Nursing ethics. 4. Nurse and patient. I.
Falk, Gerhard, 1924- II. Title.

  RT85.6.F35 2006
  610.73--dc22
                                                                    2006043313

hors série.

A CIP catalog record for this book is available from the British Library.

The Edwin Mellen Press   The Edwin Mellen Press
Box 450   Box 67
Lewiston, New York   Queenston, Ontario
USA 14092-0450   CANADA L0S 1L0

The Edwin Mellen Press, Ltd.
Lampeter, Ceredigion, Wales
UNITED KINGDOM SA48 8LT

Printed in the United States of America

This Book is dedicated to the large majority of nurses who are trustworthy, conscientious, caring; to our son Clifford. Jonathan who is always there when needed to help us with the vagaries and glitches of the computer and to our grandchildren and their mother who are our future.

Table of Contents

Chapter I

Introduction – The Nature of Deviance

Deviance Defined

Nearly half a century ago, Dentler and Erikson defined social deviance as "behavior which violates institutionalized expectations, that is, expectations which are shared and recognized as legitimate within the social system."[1]

Since then there have been several major developments in the sociological study of deviance. First we need to understand that sociologists have never acceded to the view that some acts are inherently deviant. Instead, sociologists have resorted to labeling theory which holds that an act is deviant only if so labeled. The major proponents of that view have been Kai T. Erikson and Howard Becker. Erikson defines deviance as "conduct which is generally thought to require the attention of social control agencies" so that deviance is a form of conduct upon which the label deviance is "conferred . . . by the audiences which . . . witness them."[2]

It is the further argument of Erikson as it was of Durkheim a century ago, that deviance functions to promote group cohesion. Here we once more cite the famous passage from *The Rules of the Sociological Method* in which Durkheim wrote: "Imagine a society of saints, a perfect cloister of exemplary individuals. Crimes, (deviance) properly so called will there be unknown; but faults which appear venial to the layman will create there the same scandal that the ordinary offense does in ordinary consciousnesses." Therefore, argued Durkheim, crime and deviance are functional in that they designate the limits of conduct acceptable to a group and consequently bring on social solidarity.[3]

If it is true that deviants exhibit the boundaries of group tolerance for acceptable conduct then we can see that the social system appoints some of its members to play deviant roles thereby testing the group boundaries.

In the view of Erikson, many of the institutions designed to inhibit deviance actually perpetuate deviance. This may be seen in prisons but also in hospitals because the people confined to these places interact to support one another in the deviant role they play. Alienated from the general public, the institutionalized individual can only deal with others who are also institutionalized. Therefore he learns attitudes, or skills, which perpetuate this alienation. The deviant is confronted by the community when he hears his sentence or his diagnosis which constitutes a judgment about him. Thereafter the deviant, so designated, is assigned a special role, such as prisoner or patient. Elaborate rituals are enacted to highlight the new role mandated for the deviant. A criminal trial is the most dramatic of these rituals although a lesser level of drama involves the patient assigned to a hospital and outfitted in pajamas, slippers and a robe. Because there is seldom an exit ceremony, the roles thus conferred remain with the "deviant" for some time or for the remainder of his life.

This then leads us to the "self-fulfilling prophecy." That prophecy predicts that the "deviant" will do it again, that the ex-convict will commit further crimes, that the ex-mental patient will have additional "breakdowns" and that the drug addict will never be cured. There is of course good reason to make such predictions. Numerous former offenders are involved in recidivism; many of those who have suffered psychotic episodes continue on that path later and surely very few alcoholics are ever "dry" for good. Nevertheless, the treatment accorded those who have been regarded as deviant in the past promotes deviance in the future because the outsider cannot become a trusted member of the group again and therefore is compelled to associate with other outsiders and to make his livelihood once more by stealing or prostituting or selling drugs. Therefore it is one of the insights of labeling theory that the reaction to deviance can perpetuate it so that deviance will always be with us.[4]

The Sociology of Deviance

An act is deviant if contrary to a norm. A norm is the expectation of a reference group and a reference group are all those whose views dictate the conduct of any person. For example, an orthodox Jew who associates continually with other orthodox Jews and prides himself on his orthodoxy will become a "deviant" in the eyes of his congregation if he is found to eat a pork chop at a restaurant. Yet, that same individual, eating a pork chop in the company of his Christian friends will not be viewed as a deviant at all. This illustrates that deviance depends on an audience which confers that standing on those who violate the norms of a group. It is the reaction to an act by any individual which leads to the label of deviant and not the act itself. [5]

Of course, there can be numerous reactions to any act. Therefore, a reaction to an act can be favorable and therefore avoid labeling the actor a deviant. Someone who fails to pay all the income tax demanded by the Internal Revenue Service may find that the official reaction to such a failure is negative but that many citizens applaud such conduct or at least are neutral in their reaction if they should become aware of it at all. This is further illustrated by the arrest and even conviction of innocent persons. Here we have an official designation of "criminal deviant" concerning a person who has offended no one and is yet labeled deviant.

We ask then, "what kind of reaction is necessary to designate someone as deviant?" Usually the reaction to acts deemed deviant is the use of words that are associated with being different or criminal or ill. Such words include "queer," "nut case," "pervert" "dangerous" etc. There is of course no end to such a list so that the perception and the label conferred by others largely determine who is deviant.

Since a good number of deviant acts go unpunished and even unnoticed it is doubtful whether reaction to deviant acts constitutes deviance. It has even been observed that illness is only so understood if the person who is ill accepts that label from a medical professional. People who have all kinds of physical problems but do not visit a physician, nurse etc. are considered well enough to go to work and avoid the label of "patient." Yet, there are numerous patients in doctors' offices every day who have no physical ailment but seek emotional resolutions.

Whether an act is deviant depends then on its meaning. Some acts are so regularly and commonly viewed as deviant that there is no doubt about their meaning. Robbery is an example. Surely, few if any members of any community would not regard robbery as a threat to everyone so that robbery is always and everywhere seen as offensive and means that there is danger to be anticipated on the part of robbers (deviants).

Of course, sociologists actually rely on reactive formulations concerning deviance. By using FBI statistics such as the Uniform Crime Report, sociologists confirm that official reactions to some kinds of conduct are the defining criteria of deviance. This assumes that official reactive data concerning deviance is the same or at least reflects the true extent of deviance in any community.[6]

There are then two kinds of deviant acts. Those that are contrary to norms or expectations by a reference group and those that provoke reaction leading to labeling of the individual as deviant.

In 1938, Robert K. Merton (Meyer Scholnick) proposed a theory of deviance which became immensely influential among sociologists. Merton proposed that Durkheim's phrase *anomie* explains a good deal of deviance. Durkheim had shown that any kind of disturbance in the social order increased the suicide rate so that a stock market crash as well as a sudden increase in prosperity both caused an increase in suicide. These and other examples led Durkheim and Merton to the conclusion that disruptions in the social order result in deviance.

Merton concluded that there are pressures in conventional social conditions which lead to unconventional behavior.[7]

Merton redefined Durkheim's conception of *anomie*. Instead of Durkheim's assertion that confusion of norms and too weak attachments to available norms leads to deviance, Merton asserts that too strong an attachment to available norms creates deviance. His proposal was that the disjunction between culturally defined goals and structurally available opportunities leads to deviance such as delinquency. Merton argued that almost everyone in a society shares the same goals such as gaining a great deal of money. That greed is created by the culture, said Merton, so that those who cannot attain what the culture demands because economics will not allow it, become deviant. Being affluent is no doubt the most important American goal. The means of acquiring wealth are however, not equally attainable by everyone.

Merton claimed that in contemporary America "winning at any cost" is approved by almost everyone so that legitimate avenues of attaining wealth are in competition with illegitimate means of gaining affluence. Therefore, the culture dictates that deviant means are just as acceptable as legitimate means so long as the goal, money, is attained. The basic question therefore is: "Which of the available procedures is most efficient in netting the culturally approved values?"[8]

According to Merton, the aspirations of the American population are unlimited although the chances of success are quite limited. Therefore we have a great deal of pressure to commit deviance.

Of course Merton recognized that despite these pressures to deviate, a large number of Americans are conformists who use conventionalized means of reaching desired goals. These conformists are in the majority even among those who never reach the goals they seek. Merton also proposed that there are among us numerous innovators. Those who use innovation are most likely to become deviants because they have assimilated the cultural value of the goal but do not use conventional means of achieving it. Instead they use such criminal activities as "money laundering," embezzlement, pick pocketing, robbery, burglary, prostitution etc.[9]

Over several generations Edwin Sutherland's theory of *differential association* has had some following among students of deviance. Sutherland's view of crime, or deviance, is based on the assumption that crime is learned in interaction with other persons in a process of communication. Sutherland further concluded that the principal part of the learning of criminal behavior occurs within intimate groups. In those groups the learning includes techniques of committing the crime and learning the attitude, rationalizations and motives promoting a favorable criminal definition towards violating the law. This is the essence of differential association which, according to Sutherland may vary in frequency, duration, priority and intensity. The process of learning criminal or deviant behavior involves all of the mechanism that are involved in any learning. Finally, Sutherland cautions that both deviant and non-deviant behavior are an expression of needs and values, deviance cannot be explained solely by needs and values.[10]

Sutherland's theory has been subject to a great deal of criticism and repeatedly described as not provable.

A third theory of deviance, at one time highly regarded, is sub cultural theory as promoted by Albert Cohen. Cohen saw delinquent sub-cultures as a system of beliefs and values brought about by verbal interaction among young men in similar circumstances. That value similarity is the result, according to Cohen, of similar positions in the social system. Cohen sees the subculture as a solution to the problem of adjustment to which the establishment provides no satisfactory solutions. Cohen wrote: "The delinquent sub-culture, with its characteristics of non-utilitarianism, malice and negativism, provides an alternative status system and justifies, for those who participate in it, hostility and aggression against the source of their status frustration."[11]

Cohen's and other sub cultural theories were based on the view that delinquency and other forms of deviance are concentrated in the urban lower economic sector of American society. However, self-reports concerning deviant behavior has shown that delinquency is widespread in rural areas and among suburban children including females. There is also a great deal of non-gang delinquency.

Therefore, it has become necessary to discover alternatives to subculture theories of delinquency and deviance.

The theories concerning deviance so far reviewed rely almost entirely on criminal statistics as reported in Uniform Crime Reports or Bureau of Justice

Statistics. Therefore deviance becomes dependent on the interpretation of officials. Such statistics are unreliable not only because officials may or may nor know how to deal with statistical information, but also because so much deviance is never reported to officials, whatever their competence.

Consequently, self report studies and victimization surveys have been developed to offset the limitations of "official" reports of deviance. The self report studies ask participant to anonymously report such delinquencies or crimes in which the respondent was involved. Victimization surveys are just that. They result in looking at delinquency "from the other side." Both of these methods have shown that crime and delinquency are much more common than official statistics would indicate. Such data are of course also disputable because there is no way of discovering whether or not anonymous data are reliable. Furthermore, delinquency and crime involve legal definitions which may not be known to the reporting population. It is entirely possible that someone will report having committed a crime when his conduct was in fact not a crime and not illegal. There are also crimes which have no victim such as drug use.

Finally, there are many people who will not participate in any self report study or a victimization survey so that a sample is not likely to be accurate.

In 1972, Edwin Lemert pointed out that "secondary deviance refers to a class of socially responses which people make to problems created by the societal reaction to their deviance." [12]

This means that those who behave in a manner usually labeled deviant, such as drug addicts, ex-convicts, alcoholics, prostitutes are expected to conduct themselves in a fashion that corresponds to the label attached to their deviance. Hence, the deviant is shunned, distrusted and excluded from normal social relations. This treatment in turn causes the "deviant" to view himself as deviant with the result that more deviant action will be undertaken by the person so labeled. That is the meaning of secondary deviance. This is also called "stigma" and refers to the role the stigmatized person is forced to accept because he is offered no alternatives. The individual so treated will play the role of deviant because the deviant has little choice but to adapt to the role assigned to him. [13]

It should not be ignored that there are of course many individuals who do not accept the role of deviant even if the reaction to their deviant conduct is negative. Therefore, only some deviants may become "secondary" deviants in so far as they accept the label placed on them.

There are two classifications of theories of deviance. These consist of those that emphasize generative conditions such as unemployment or drug addiction and those that emphasize inhibiting conditions such as legal punishments. These are called "social control" theories.

Social control rests on the assumption that some kinds of behavior are "bad" and that therefore such behavior needs to be kept in check by the agents of social control such as police, clergy, teachers etc. These agents of social control seek to suppress deviance by defining the deviant as evil and thereby elevating the members of the larger society to the status of "good" and superior. This in turn allows the "good" members of a society to feel a sense of solidarity in view of the "evil" outcast who becomes the subject of any methods the agents of social control may wish to use against him. Police are the best examples of social control agents in American society. Therefore police are also the best example of escalation in that police are often the party responsible for another's violence, making police the cause of deviance. Examples are family disturbances which are escalated by police intervention to become far more serious than they were before police intervened. Riot control is another example of police escalation of deviance. The best example of that were the riots by the Chicago police themselves during the 1968 Democratic convention in that city. That example also serves to illustrate an increase in the frequency of deviance produced by efforts to control the deviance. In addition, efforts to control deviance often lead to the advent of new categories of deviants. High speed chases originating with the police can result in injury and death which are then attributed to the traffic violator who only became involved in these tragic forms of deviance because the police chased him. The real cause of these form of "crimes" is denial of police authority.

An even more egregious form of deviance are crimes created by the agents of social control. The imprisonment of Martha Stewart for lying to an investigator is an excellent example of this form of "deviance." Stewart was never charged with stock fraud or insider trading because this could not be proved. Failing to find such deviant conduct on her part, government bureaucrats jailed her for "obstruction of justice" which has no secure definition and can be used to jail any citizen merely by defining any opinion as an "obstruction of justice." Here the agents of social control actually create the crime.

A further example of government created "crime" is the lengthening of prison sentences for those prisoners who are sent to prison for a short time but have their sentences constantly increased because of rule violations within the prison.[14]

Not only agencies of social control, but also self-rejection can lead to deviance. Deviance usually reflects a violation of internalized values, except for a minority who have no conscience. Furthermore, deviance evokes rejection by other group members. That rejection in turn leads to self rejection subsequent to social exclusion.[15]

Applying these views to the deviant nurses described in this book, we see that deviance among nurses follows the same sociological patterns visible in all deviants. Therefore, it would be unrealistic to expect only normative individuals in the nursing profession despite training and supervision. All professions must deal with those who deviate from its ideals and the expectations of their clients and nursing is no exception.

Notes

1. Robert A. Dentler and Kai T. Erikson, " The Functions of Deviance in Groups," *Social Problems*, 7(Fall 1959):98-107.

2. Kai T. Erikson, "Notes on the Sociology of Deviance," *Social Problems*, 9, (1962):307-314.

3. Emile Durkheim, "The Normal and the Pathological," in: Henry N. Potell, editor, *Social Deviance*, (Upper Saddle River, N.J. Pearson, Prentice Hall, 2005):36.

4. Harold Garfinkel, "Successful Degradation Ceremonies," *American Journal of Sociology*,61, (1956): 420-424.

5. Jack P. Gibbs and Maynard J. Erickson, "Major Developments in the Sociological Study of Deviance," *Annual Review of Sociology*, 1, (1975):21-42.

6. Ibid. p. 23.

7. Robert K. Merton, "Social Structure and Anomie," *American Sociological Review*, 3, (October 1938):672-682.

8. Robert K. Merton, *Social Theory and Social Structure*, (New York: Free Press, 1957)p. 135.

9. Merton, *Social Structure*, 180.

10. Edwin H. Sutherland, Donald R. Cressey and David F. Luckenbill, *Principles of Criminology*, (Dix Hills, N.Y. 1992)p.88-92.

11. Albert K. Cohen and James F. Short, Jr. , "Research in Delinquent Sub-cultures," *Journal of Social Issues*, 14, (1958):20.

12. Edwin M. Lemert, *Human Deviance, Social Problems and Social Control*, (Englewood Cliffs, N.J., Prentice-Hall, 1967)pp.17. 60.

13. Gerhard Falk, *Stigma: How We Treat Outsiders*, (Amherst, N.Y. Prometheus Books, 2001) p.11.

14. Gary T. Marx, "Ironies of Social Control," *Social Problems*, 28:3 (February 1981):221-233.

15. Howard B. Kaplan, Robert J. Johnson and Carol A. Bailey, "Self-rejection and the explanation of deviance," *Social Psychology Quarterly*, 49, no.2, (June 1986): 110.

Chapter II

The Caring Profession – Nursing the Sick

It must be remembered that the large majority of nurses give of themselves unstintingly to countless patients who are in pain, both physically and emotionally. They know the true meaning of serving with love.

When you are admitted to a hospital or enter a nursing home do you know who is taking care of you? Are they nurses, are they responsible, knowledgeable, what are their credentials, are they honorable, have they committed a felony or two and who are they?

There were 1,908,470 registered nurses (RN's) in the United States in 1998 as reported on March 12th of that year by the U.S. Bureau of Labor Statistics.

Of these 27,000 are in the State of New York There are the Registered Professional Nurses as well as the Licensed Practical Nurses. Most of the women and men who enter this profession are caring, honest and hardworking people.

They entered into this honorable occupation because they wanted to serve people, to help humanity – one person at a time. Their training included not only academics but the practical aspects of carrying out their chosen field. They learned to make beds, dress wounds, assist in emergency rooms, handing instruments to surgeons, sterilizing equipment, ascertaining that infection control is adhered to in the most scrupulous sense, giving injections, extracting blood samples, inserting intravenous lines, operating oxygen equipment, attaching nasal tubes, disimpacting anal cavities, performing Heimlich maneuvers, distributing medications, documenting patients conditions, observations of same, comforting the frightened and sick and much, much more.

The tasks of the nurse are almost limitless, their observational and hands on skills must be great, their ability to read and take physicians orders essential and their memory good. Their hands must be impeccably clean, their scrubbing techniques beyond reproach; their handwriting legible. They must know how to transfer, lift and turn, to teach these techniques to the nurses aides, to remain calm under crisis conditions, to be attentive to their charges and to work hard and fast. The ideal nurse must be able to get along with people, must not overstep her bounds, must be diplomatic and soothing at all times, must be able to give and take orders, must be able to dispense medication accurately and in a timely fashion. She must never leave her shift or her patients under any circumstance until her replacement appears.

Who are these Florence Nightingales? What are their backgrounds, their personalities, their goals, their objectives? What are their needs, their desires, their abilities? How are they trained and educated? What does their curriculum consist of? What are their opportunities for employment, how do they view themselves, their colleagues, their peers, their patients and their responsibilities? How are they similar or different from each other and from folks in other professions or careers?

All of these factors must be viewed in order to enable us to know and to understand what nursing in the twenty-first century entails and why, how and not infrequently, the unexpected happens.

A registered nurse is one who has passed the national licensing examination known as the State Board Test Pool. This examination became nation-wide in 1950 when all U.S. States and some Canadian provinces adopted the same examination as a means of obtaining nursing licensure and registration.[1]

The income of nurses varies widely because the responsibilities of nurses range over such a large area of work. Anesthesiology nurses earned an average salary of $73,756 in 1997 but a "head nurse" and all others earned a good deal less than that. "Head nurses" received an average of $47,270 in 1997, "charge nurses" earned an average salary of $42,480, "staff nurses" earned $41,704, "operating room nurses" $41,412, intensive care nurses" $40,435, "medical-surgical nurses," $39,499 and "emergency room" nurses $39, 062. It is evident from this list that the median annual earnings of registered nurses, $36,244 is less than half of the average salary earned by anesthesiology nurses. It is also noteworthy that male nurses earn five percent more than women, who constituted 94 percent of the membership in that profession in 1997.[2]

The earnings of Licensed Practical Nurses are a good deal less. Typical of the education of LPNs is the law in the State of Washington requiring 450 hours of special preparation and 5 months on-the-job training to attain a practical nurse license.[3] The earnings of licensed practical nurses reflect this difference in training. The median income of the 640,000 American LPNs was $25,000 a year or 69 percent of the median earnings of registered nurses in 1997. [4]

The licensing of registered and practical nurses is now only a half a century old. Its original purpose was not only to protect the public but also to give nurses and other licensed professions the independence a license implies. Yet, now, at the end of five decades of government regulated licensure, a number of states have proposed the disbanding of regulatory boards to allow unlicensed workers to provide at least some home and community services. The consequence of that procedure must be that without government controls, oversight falls to the employer, making that method a *de facto* institutional licensure. Such a trend would return the nursing professions to the time before 1950 when nurses were viewed as having primary responsibility to the employer and not the patient. The license reversed that approach and allowed nurses to be more responsive to the needs of the patient than the financial interests of institutions. In view of the tremendous drive to lower costs of medical care underway at the end of this century it is almost certain that institutional licensure will sacrifice the interests of the patient to the financial advantages of hospital administrators. Obviously, nurses would not be free to speak out in favor of patients if their employer is also the regulator. This demonstrates that financial interests so dominate the American health delivery system that Hippocrates has indeed been assailed if not betrayed and that every level of health care is about to be "dumbed down" to save money. [5]

Even as nurses are concerned about the gradual encroachment of unlicensed and untrained personnel into their area of expertise, nurses themselves are entering the practice of medicine on the grounds that they know as much about the treatment of patients as any graduate of a medical school. Convinced that this is so, 52 percent of patients surveyed in 1998 were "very willing" to see a registered nurse rather than a physician. If it is true that nurse-practitioners can function like doctors of medicine with only five years of schooling past high school, then it becomes legitimate to ask: "Why should the medical education of primary care physicians take in excess of ten years?" There are those who would deny the need for a medical education. However, Kassirer argues that nurses cannot perform as well as physicians because nurses are not sufficiently trained to recognize a complex medical problem that "requires reasoning from first principles." We would wonder how it is possible that medical care of patients requires less training in 2000 than it did in 1980. [6]

It is therefore most likely that the effort to give nurses the responsibilities heretofore allocated to physicians is driven, once more, by financial considerations. These financial considerations are the chief concern of health maintenance organizations that have lobbied the government successfully in gaining the right of nurse-practitioners to receive reimbursement from Medicare. Medicare is only one of five basic programs under which the federal government buys health care. The others are: the Department of Defense Civilian Health and Medical Program of the Uniformed Services, the Federal Employees' Health Benefit Program, the income tax provisions subsidizing health care expenditures and Medicaid. The inclusion of nurse-practitioners among those receiving payments from Medicare was contained in the Balanced Budget Act of 1997, which Congress passed and which was signed into law in August of that year. This law extended the Community Nursing Organization pilot project until the end of 1999. Community nursing organizations are managed care programs operated by nurses. These programs offer Medicare benefits to the old in non-institutional settings, i.e. in nurses' offices. The programs are run by nurse practitioners.[7] Such nurse practitioners are also known as advanced practice registered nurses and clinical nurse specialists. Heretofore, such nurses had to either work in nursing homes or in narrowly defined rural areas. In nursing homes registered nurses have achieved dominance in decision making because doctors visit nursing homes only temporarily and because many nursing home managers have no medical or nursing training themselves. Therefore, such managers must rely on nurses for advice both on the strategic decision making level and in regard to the day-to-day, tactical type decisions.[8]

Prior to the Balanced Budget Act of 1997 those nurses who practiced outside defined rural areas had to be supervised by a physician and to be in the physical presence of a physician while administering services. Under these circumstances the supervising physicians and not the nurses billed Medicare. Therefore, the right of nurses to bill Medicare themselves will reveal the volume and the kind of services performed by nurses. Although the new Medicare law intends that nurses work in collaboration with a physician, several states, under pressure from the American Nurses Association have avoided the issue of physician collaboration. This then indicates that the emerging health delivery system in America is about to become stratified beginning with unlicensed practical nurses and ranging all the way to highly trained medical specialists whom the patient will only see after visiting the entire array of providers leading to the final diagnosis. This system is undoubtedly far more efficient than the chaos prevailing before 1995. Nevertheless, this stratified system involves the inherent danger that a patient will be permanently injured or die before a "provider" sees him who can recognize the patient's problem and deal with it.[9]

The tendency of hospitals to substitute licensed practical nurses and unlicensed assisting personnel for registered nurses, together with the introduction of nurse practitioners, has altered the future of the nurse labor market considerably. Traditionally, two thirds of all registered nurses had been employed in hospitals. However, the effort to reduce costs at any price has recently led to the substitution of licensed practical nurses for registered nurses. Likewise, changes in other areas of employment have also affected nurses in recent years. This means that there has been a shift in nursing personnel out of hospitals and into health care organizations. As hospitals have "downsized," nurses have lost their jobs. This has been most frequent in Southern California, New York and Connecticut. In those states intense competition between managed care organizations has led to hospital downsizing and a decrease in nurse employment. This decrease includes licensed practical nurses who are being replaced by aides who are now being trained, more or less, as so-called "multi-skilled workers" to reduce costs.

It remains to be seen whether these measures will really reduce costs. Because hospitals are discharging patients earlier, the need for home health care is now greater than ever before. Therefore, the use of registered and licensed nurses in home health care has risen substantially as RN's particularly use a "high-tech" approach in caring for their patients. This trend has increased the pay of nurses so that it may well be that the costs associated with the early discharge policies of hospitals will be absorbed by the home health care costs these discharges must entail. In addition, the ever growing pressure to impose a mechanistic medical model on nursing can and will result in undermining the basic values of the nursing profession. This failure to recognize the need for humanitarian caring for the sick and disabled must result in job dissatisfaction, stress and frustration and confrontations between patients, nurses and administrators. The great German sociologist Max Weber foresaw this development when he said in *The Protestant Ethic and the Spirit of Capitalism*: ." . .for the last stage of this cultural development it might well be truly said: specialists without spirit, sensualists without a heart, this nullity imagines that it has attained a level of civilization never before achieved."[10]

That word from Weber surely applies to nursing homes which have increased so much during the ten years ending in 2000. Therefore, a good number of registered nurses have indeed been absorbed into nursing homes in recent years. However, here too aides have been hired in record number to keep expenses as low as possible. The sum of all this stress on finances is of course that patients are treated mainly by untrained or under-trained health delivery workers, a situation over which the patients who need help the most have the least control.[11]

Registered nurses have traditionally been trained to work in hospitals and not in nursing homes or home health care situations. Therefore, the basic educational curriculum in nursing schools is now being changed so that future nurses will be able to practice alone. Responding to that need, the American Association of Colleges of Nursing has developed new standards for baccalaureate nursing education.[12]

The primary purpose of state legislatures in requiring a professional practitioner to hold a license is reputedly the need to protect the public. Indeed, if anyone could practice nursing without training of any kind then such a license would hardly serve a legitimate purpose. Of course, relatives and friends continue to nurse those near and dear to them at home and even in part in hospitals and nursing homes solely on grounds of love and duty. Similarly, almost everyone has given medical advice to members of his family or "practiced law" on anyone willing to listen.

Licensing is therefore an effort to protect those who pay for the services of someone who, they believe, can be trusted to know how to best meet their needs. The public, as well as legislators have evidently decided that nursing has developed sufficient clinical skills to trust its practitioners to practice on their own, i.e., to be autonomous. Additionally, universities and the profession itself have developed enough internal agreement to be able to supervise their own members and to set limits as to their competence. Practically, state legislatures become willing to enact licensing requirements when a profession has achieved enough "grass roots" support to make licensing politically feasible.[13]

This "grass roots" support was engendered by home health care nurses, who, as we have seen, have increased their importance during the past several years as admissions to hospitals have decreased and accelerated discharges have become the rule. Many patients who would have been cared for in a hospital are now receiving home health care. Therefore, nurses who were discharged from hospital jobs are now performing in home health care, although doctors do not always recognize contributions from the nursing profession. The type of knowledge and skills learned by nursing students at the baccalaureate level is of course such that it can be applied to home health care as well. Yet, there is concern that these skills and that knowledge will gradually be lost by nurses who do not see patients in the context of the hospital. Home health care places almost all of the responsibility for the patient on the shoulders of the nurse. That responsibility includes extensive documentation, i.e. "paper work." Because patients who are discharged early from hospitals after an operation need the skills of medical-surgical nurses, such nurses are sought out by home health clinics. Executives of such clinics say that it takes at least six months, if not eighteen, for an erstwhile hospital nurse to become efficient in home health care. Therefore, a program is needed which can be used to prepare acute care nurses for home health nursing demands. One such program has been developed in the State of Washington. There, nurses have listed case finding, screening, assessment, case management, a number of administrative and legal issues and a caregiver value orientation as the most important needs which should be taught to all home health nurses.[14] Numerous other proposals by a variety of administrators, writers and nurse-practitioners all agree that home health nurses should be competent in physical assessment and diagnosis and have a good knowledge of nutrition and family counseling.

In Massachusetts the American Nurses Association has developed a curriculum yielding twelve college credits towards the RN-BSN degree. Upon completion of that degree and the gaining of some experience a master's program in community health nursing is now available in many American universities and colleges. Local home health agencies, however, increasingly hire nurses with an Associates degree, i.e. a degree granted by a two year community college. Therefore, advanced degrees are usually earned by those who are already working with two years of training and who must therefore be accommodated by coming to class in the evening. Many such students have been out of school for years and need special orientation to libraries, computers and other methods not in vogue at the time of their graduation.

In Omaha, Neb. a four-fold curriculum is taught to home health care nursing students and to working nurses. This includes environment, psychosocial behavior, physiological behavior and health related behavior. The curriculum includes the study of 44 problems that are designed to "stimulate the student's awareness of the breadth of home health practice." [15]

Home health care nurses are also expected to be able to work for insurance companies and in managed care organizations. These organizations have created an "upswing" for nurses with graduate degrees. This development confirms the view that the future in the nursing profession will increasingly belong to the "advanced practice nurses" who are in fact practicing medicine. These nurses diagnose and order medicine and decide when a patient is ready to go home. Such nurses are supplanting physicians. Because this opportunity to practice medicine without having to undergo the rigors of a medical school education is so attractive, enrollment in master's degree programs at nursing schools has risen by nearly 2 percent each year since 1996. Enrollment at bachelor's level programs fell by nearly 7 percent during the same years. Consequently, the number of universities offering programs for nurse practitioners have also increased. In 1992 there were 119 such programs. At the end of 1997 there were 202 with more in preparation. Acute care specialization has also increased so that 26 schools offered training in that specialty at the end of 1997 while only one such program existed in 1992 at the University of Pennsylvania. Here students are taught how to make decisions concerning treatment, drug therapy and the use of appropriate technology. Students in such programs are generally registered nurses with eight to nine years experience. Because the kinds of programs offered by different universities vary so much in requirements and in faculty preparation the Commission on Collegiate Nursing Education has published criteria designed to standardize such programs. [16]

One such program was instituted at Syracuse University's school of nursing. It is one of the schools offering a master's degree for a nurse practitioner. This costs $20,000 while a graduate certificate program in the same specialty costs the student $8,000.- Because of these high costs and because of the intense and difficult course work needed to attain such a degree, students who had already spent a year in the program were shocked to learn in August of 1998 that Syracuse University had never received New York State certification to operate such a program. Twenty two students were affected by the failure of the dean of nursing to tell them that the state had three times turned down the Syracuse University proposal to certify the family nurse-practitioner program. The state Education Department refused to do so because of a lack of faculty qualifications as family nurse-practitioners. Evidently, the administration of the university concealed this information from the students because they did not want to lose thousands of dollars of federal funding that came with those students.[17] State certification seeks to assure that advanced practice nurses are trained to conduct physical examinations, diagnose and treat minor illnesses and injuries, order lab tests and X-rays and interpret results, and counsel patients. Advanced practice nurses are now also preferred by women who need "colposcopy," which is a visual examination of the cervix to discover the possibility of cancer. In view of the many tasks nurses have now undertaken it is significant that a recent review of 210 studies comparing the care given by doctors and nurses found that nurses perform as well as physicians. Nevertheless, it must be remembered that nurses do not possess a medical education and may have difficulty diagnosing ambiguous symptoms.[18]

Community health nurses may be private practitioners. Others have entered the field of public health nurse. In that capacity nurses seek to compete with social workers and with doctors, particularly in rural communities. In such communities patients are often more sick and in need of more services than is true in cities. This is so because of early patient discharge, short hospital stays, increased "ambulatory" care and home health care.[19]

Technology has also given community health nurses an opportunity to enter into areas of care once reserved for the hands of physicians. Intravenous therapy, wound irrigation, respirators used at home by patients and other devices are now the province of nurses. Nurses also counsel family caregivers, particularly in hospices and in other settings among the terminally ill. This situation is particularly acute with the growing number of AIDS patients as AIDS has reached epidemic proportions in this country.

Because acquired immune deficiency syndrome is a transmissible and is frequently a fatal disease, nurses rightly perceive a personal vulnerability in caring for such AIDS patients. This means that nurses who work with AIDS patients are likely to suffer an increase in death anxiety leading to avoidance, extreme precautions and a lack of regard for those suffering from the disease. It is therefore in the interest of dying patients and the nursing profession if means could be found that can overcome death anxiety. Such means can be a greater awareness of ourselves as members of a group of family and friends. That kind of awareness has the merit of calling attention to the endless continuity of life and therefore reduces death anxiety. Furthermore, those who hold some fundamental values, be they of a religious or philosophical nature, are also less anxious about death or non-being. Death can be given meaning by such a set of values, particularly if we have some important life goals that we are working to fulfill. Surely, the care of the sick and the dying can be such a life goal. Hence, nurses who care for AIDS patients can be induced to recognize the importance of their work and the meaning their work gives their lives. There are of course those who interpret death as punishment and who fear going "to hell" and suffering unpleasant cruelties after death. Such notions certainly heighten death anxiety. There are innumerable explanations for death anxiety, ranging from Freud's view that death anxiety is really a fear of castration and separation anxiety. There are others who seek the cause of death anxiety in deprivation in the mother-child relationship; as loss of control and fear of pain. There are many other "explanations." It has been proposed that those who view themselves as more than a physical body can accept death without fear because they see death as part of life. Such an attitude can view death as another form of being outside the body and without bodily constraints in which the self does not cease to exist. Because Americans principally interpret the world in purely physical terms, death anxiety can be high among the religious as well as the non religious segment of the American population. Religious conduct consists of participation in ritual and therefore has visible and physical aspects. It is however awareness of our connection to the universe that permits us to recognize our co-existence with other living things which reduces death anxiety and confronts the view that death is final or even absolute. In fact, in the Buddhist and Hindu tradition death is viewed as liberation and hence can be confronted without fear. This view is of course open to anyone and is not confined to the Hindu-Buddhist tradition.[20]

Finally, a high exposure to death also reduces death-anxiety although Americans are seldom present at someone's death as are nurses.[21]

Nurses are far more likely to be caring for dying patients than is true of doctors. Therefore nursing educators have been interested in teaching nursing students how to provide physical, emotional and spiritual support to the dying patient and his family. Beck reports on the feelings of nursing students as they came to deal with the imminent death of their patients. According to that report, nursing students generally experienced one or more of six reactions as a consequence of dealing with dying patients. Initially students experienced fear. Later they became more comfortable with their feelings towards the dying although many sought to emotionally distance themselves from the dying patient and his family. Many nursing students, as well as many people everywhere, believe that they lack the right words to use in face of death and therefore feel uncomfortable discussing death. Many nursing students, as well as others, also feel anger at physicians for not doing more for the dying patients. A second reaction of nursing students to their dying patients was contemplation of the dying patient's life and the kind of life that patient had led. Thirdly, nursing students realized that the dying patient's family became part of their responsibility as well. The grieving family is evidently very much in need of support so that a nurse will have to decide how to divide her time between the dying patient and the family. Nurses and nursing students also feel helpless in giving the dying patient more pain medication and in carrying out the dying patient's last wishes. Often nurses know these wishes better than family who may not be present when such wishes are made. Nursing students and others also learn that holding a dying person's hand and speaking or praying with the dying patient is most useful in providing comfort to the dying. Discussing the patient's imminent death is essential in such a situation as the fear of dying ebbs and flows in such patients. The sixth and most important lesson nursing students learned was that unconditional and non-judgmental caring helps not only those who eventually get well but also helps those who die. This illustrates that the help anyone can give the dying is not wasted but of great importance.[22]

It is of course on that principle that the hospice movement was founded by Cicely Saunders in London, England. The first hospice in the United States was established in Branford, Connecticut in 1974. Today there are 3,000 hospice programs in this country serving 450,000 patients at any one time. Currently these programs are growing at the rate of 17 percent annually.[23]

No conclusive research concerning these hospices exists now. The National Hospice Organization does have a survey asking families to report their satisfaction with the outcome of hospice care and that appears to be positive. However, the health maintenance organizations, in their anxiety to make money, have minimized the emotional and spiritual care which was the basis for the hospice movement at the outset. That beginning occurred in London, England in 1967 when the first residential hospice was opened in that city. Initially, hospices were supported by religious groups who did not charge their patients. These constitute about 20 percent of American hospices. Thereafter, secular community based organizations initiated about 28 percent of American hospices while hospitals support another 28 percent. Nineteen percent of hospices are divisions of home health care agencies, 6 percent are hospice corporations and one percent are divisions of nursing homes. Another eighteen percent of hospices are privately owned. Michael Sorrow, director of Southwest Christian Hospice, has said that "Once Medicare and Medicaid came out with the benefit, every Tom, Dick and Harry jumped into the hospice business to make money on it." Likewise, Jack Gordon, president of the Hospice Foundation of America accuses the HMO's of refusing to pay for bereavement care "because after the patient is dead they don't want to spend any money." No doubt, the "Business First" attitude of the HMOs has deprived the hospice movement of much of its reason for existence in limiting the care given patients and survivors. The HMOs want the clergy to deal with the dying for free because they don't want to pay social workers and nurses. They seek to cut the cost of care below the Medicare and Medicaid reimbursement rate in order to profit from the difference between costs and income. This was possible because heretofore Medicaid and Medicare paid a flat daily rate no matter how much or how little service was rendered the patient. Evidently, this system leads to minimizing the amount of service given the dying although Medicaid and Medicare have also enlarged the number of dying patients to whom hospice care can be made available.

In November of 1997, Oregon became the first state to permit physician-assisted suicide. Thereupon the health maintenance organizations began to lobby for such laws in all other states because their profits increase as patients die sooner. Because assisted suicide is cheaper, HMOs and insurance companies favor hospices which allow assisted suicide.

There are now 2,154 hospices in the United States. In 1997 Medicaid paid $94 a day for home care and $419 for general inpatient care to the eighty percent of hospices now Medicare certified. More than 90 percent of hospice care occurs in patients' homes and is generally administered by nurses.[24]

The care of the old living in the community is another function assigned to public health nurses. This interest has become most important in recent years as the American population has lived to a greater age and as the emphasis in nursing has shifted from acute care to prevention. Nurses dealing with the old must of course be well informed about chronic illness with particular reference to cardiovascular and pulmonary conditions.

Such nurses may be called "geriatric nurse practitioners." These specialists can help the old maintain their independence and lower the chance that they will have to go to a nursing home. This view is supported by a three year controlled study of more than 400 senior citizens with an average age of 81 and living at home when the study began. This study concluded that at the end of three years the study subjects were 60 percent less likely than the control group to need assistance with the most basic activities of daily living such as bathing, dressing and moving about the house. As a consequence there was also a 60 percent decline in the chance of the study subjects moving into a nursing home during the three years involved.[25]

Community nurses are of course concerned with patients "from the cradle to the grave." Therefore, such nurses are also engaged in baby and child care, particularly because there are numerous rural counties in America which have no medical resources other than a public health nurse. For example, in Alabama 26 out of 67 counties have no obstetrical services other than a public health nurse. These nurses live in generally inaccessible areas and therefore find it difficult to participate in continuing education available only at colleges and universities in larger communities.

In a national survey, Stevens and Silverman found that 76 percent of their respondents said that no continuing education was available in their area for non-BSN community health nurses. In view of the foregoing discussion of the numerous responsibilities of such nurses it is evident that telecommunications classes wold be the only means of reaching such nurses. Unfortunately, such classes are now available in only 50 percent of the states. [26]

Because nurses have become heavily involved in the delivery of babies, known as midwifery, education for this profession is provided at various universities at the graduate level for those nursing students who have passed a certification examination. Today, in 1999, certified nurse midwives are autonomous patient care providers. They provide prenatal care, labor and delivery management, well-woman gynecology, normal newborn care, and family planning. Certified nurse midwives now also have prescription authority. There are about 5,200 certified nurse midwives in the U.S. In addition to private practice they are found in community clinics and sponsored health care programs. In recent years they have accounted for 196,225 American births or about five percent of all U.S. deliveries.[27]

Brown and Grimes report that in more than 50 studies nurse midwives have shown themselves to be the equals of doctors in the delivery of pre-natal and natal care. According to these 50 studies, C-section, fetal distress and neo-natal mortality rates were the same whether treated by a physician or a nurse. [28]

Another area of child nursing which has traditionally been the exclusive domain of registered nurses is school nursing. This is an aspect of independent nursing which has long been accepted by the public.[29]

In 1998, the Health Resources and Services Administration of the U.S. Public Health Service contracted with the American Association of Colleges of Nursing to determine how nurse practitioners, certified nurse midwives and physician assistants can be used to meet health care needs in underserved areas in the United States. Such a contractual arrangement is important to Americans living in rural areas because the National Health Services Corps is the only source of health care for many Americans. Under the four- month contract the American Association of Colleges of Nursing will evaluate the availability of health care in rural locations and will also report the specialties of health care providers in such areas. The purpose is evidently to determine which clinics are eligible for Federal funding and to provide scholarships and educational loan programs to attract nursing and other health professions students to the National Health Services Corps.[30]

The need for new methods and new curricula in training nurses is determined by the evolution of nursing into a technologically sophisticated practice discipline. This may not be the choice of nurses themselves. Yet, advances in electrophysiological monitoring systems, computerized surgical techniques and integrated hospital information systems force nurses to become proficient in the use of computer technology as well as the traditional practice of nursing. The development of nursing technology is called "informatics" and has become the newest field of nursing specialization. Nursing "informatics" combines computer information and nursing sciences. Most Americans, whether in nursing or not, are of course at least somewhat acquainted with the use of computers which are already installed in almost all grade schools in America. Nevertheless, about 30 percent of nurses report that they are uncomfortable with computers, are intimidated by computers or have had no experience with them.[31]

The outcome of the ever-increasing use of technology in nursing is, hopefully, greater productivity and efficiency on behalf of the patient without losing sight of the patient's emotional, social and spiritual needs. Therefore, it is recommended that nurses investigate more carefully the stories patients tell about their hospital experiences. Such investigation will reveal that many patients have had negative experiences in hospitals and other treatment centers but are given no opportunity to discuss these feelings with nurses.[32]

The reason for failure to give patients experiences much credence, is that researchers have limited their information to those areas of knowledge which concern them. They view themselves as "experts" and seek to determine what is or is not information. Yet, patients are in fact the real "experts" concerning their treatment so that research methodology must include the patient if it is to be valid.[33]

Another consequence of the many changes in the nursing profession at the end of the twentieth century is the need to delegate many erstwhile nursing responsibilities to nonprofessional personnel who deliver patient care. There are a number of reasons for this need to delegate. First among these reasons is the unwillingness of hospitals to employ a sufficient number of registered nurses despite the availability of such nurses. Evidently, the few registered nurses who are employed cannot do everything themselves, not only because of time limitations but also because "short cuts" and haste can put patients at risk. The early discharge programs mandated by health maintenance organizations; advanced technology and the ever - increasing demand for patient's rights are additional reasons for the need to delegate nurses' tasks to others. Such delegation can involve a risk to the patient and can also lead to legal liability to the hospital and the nurse if the patient is injured or maltreated because a nonprofessional was empowered to treat a patient. Not only is it possible for a non-professional to perform a task incorrectly, but non-professionals are less likely to recognize a change in a patient's status than is true of professionals.[34]

Despite these threats to the well-being of hospitalized patients, some health-care facilities are "cross training" janitors, housekeepers, security guards and aides and "multi-skilled" workers who are assigned to nursing duties. This "cross-training" may range from a few hours to six weeks. Few hospitals require a high school diploma from those now involved in such "cross-training" and hence responsiblity for the well being of patients. Patients are of course not only concerned with pills and instruments but with their survival and the administration of life support.

The phrase "life support" is readily identified as a series of technological inventions such as mechanical ventilators, dialysis machines, intravenous pumps, biomedical research, surgery and medication. These physical methods are undoubtedly important in permitting the survival of many patients who would have died if these contrivances were not available. There is however one more life support available in our health delivery system. That life support is the 2.2 million nurses who are the second largest profession, after teaching, in the United States. Staffed almost, but not entirely, by women "these women and men weave a tapestry of care, knowledge and trust that is critical to patients' survival."[35]

Because cost-cutting is the most important motive driving hospital and insurance administrators, American hospitals are already using 20 percent fewer nurses than is the case in other industrialized nations. Despite the fact that nurses cost only 16 percent of hospital expenditures, many hospitals are planning to reduce their nursing staff up to 50 percent.

As the cost-cutting epidemic has reduced the number of competent nurses greatly, those who are still employed are now forced to spend almost all their time writing reports and "documenting" each patient endlessly. As a result, patients can hardly expect to be seen by the limited number of registered nurses still available as their economic security and professional career depends on what they write and not whom they nurse.

We have already seen that the median salary of nurses in 1998 was approximately $36,000. Physicians earn about four times more. The highest earnings among those working in hospitals or anywhere in the health delivery system does not go to physicians but to the so-called "bean counters," i.e. executives interested in the business aspects of health care. A recent survey of executive salaries in health care revealed that the average total cash compensation of hospital executives is $188,500 and that large hospitals pay as much as $281,000 annual salary. For-profit health maintenance organizations pay yet more. Richard Scott, chief executive officer of Columbia Health Care Corporation received more than $2 million in 1996. The seven largest for-profit health maintenance organizations paid their CEOs an average of $7 million.

The immense salary discrepancy between the compensation given nurses and the compensation given doctors and business managers in health care represent the value placed on the work of each profession in the eyes of the American public. Income reflects status in America. Men constituted only seven percent of all American nurses at the end of this century. Hence nursing is mainly a female profession and is therefore devalued so that nursing pays less than do other aspects of the health related professions dominated by men. This discrepancy is gradually lessening but is nevertheless very much in force.[36]

There is an additional reason for the devaluation of nursing in comparison to the practice of medicine and the practice of accounting in the health delivery system. That reason is the devaluation of the work that nurses do. In part, that devaluation is contingent on the belief that anyone can nurse because everyone has on numerous occasions nursed children and relatives at home. Furthermore, nurses work frequently goes unrecognized because they remind us of our failure to be in control. Nursing reminds us of our pain, of our fears, of our worst moments. Indeed, nurses are now more than ever competent to use the most sophisticated technology. Yet, we attribute sophistication and knowledge to doctors and minimize the help derived from our nurses who may clean our most intimate areas one minute and administer our medicine the next. All this is viewed in the nursing profession as evidence that caring for the patient is still the most important task of the nurse.[37]

Because the nursing profession has always maintained that caring is their most important task, emphasis on caring has evolved into the profession's subculture. Every occupation is a sub-culture. This means that every occupation includes fundamental attitudes, values and beliefs which define the work the occupation demands of its practitioners. This is true of nursing as well as it is true of other occupations and professions. We have seen that nursing has changed a great deal in recent years and that therefore cost containment, technology and its attendant bureaucracy have all militated against caring for patients as people.

Nursing surely seeks to strive for independence from the medical profession and to create a unique place for itself in the conglomerate of health delivery systems. Therefore it is of the utmost importance that nursing continue in the tradition of caring for the patient even as more and more radical changes are occurring in the intellectual development, training and education of the profession.

These changes are visible if we examine the trends in nursing education which have occurred during the past thirty years. Thus, in 1965 eighty percent of all new nurse graduates were trained in hospital diploma programs. After 1988, less than 12 percent of new graduates came from hospital diploma programs while the vast majority graduated from college and university four-year programs. Included in any form of education for nursing is clinical practice that is generally undertaken by clinical teachers on the staff of the university. Such practice must of necessity occur in a hospital so that a division develops between the classroom education and the "hands-on" education provided by clinical teachers in the territory of the hospital nurses. Paterson has described the experiences of clinical nursing teachers in such a hospital setting. She shows that success in providing a clinical education to students depends largely on an understanding of the relationship of temporary systems to permanent systems in the negotiated order of the hospital.[38]

A temporary system in a work situation can be auditors, researchers involved in a temporary research project or politically appointed task forces. Likewise, clinical teachers and their students are a temporary system intruding on the routine of the permanent system. According to Paterson, the language used by permanent staff concerning clinical teachers and their students reveals a real division of territory between the temporary outsiders and the regular nursing staff. Even the language used by regular staff concerning students differs from the language used by students and their clinical teachers. Staff refer to "your students" when addressing clinical teachers. They talk about "our conference room" and "our medication room" and view the presence of students not as an opportunity to teach but as help with their workload. These attitudes result in an "us against them" situation for both clinical teachers and staff nurses and has as a consequence that many clinical teachers cannot carry out their ideas of how to train nursing students in hospitals. Defensiveness, territoriality and separateness all militate against the nurse student and finally against the patient.[39]

It has become customary now to train medical students, nurse students, pharmacy students and physical therapy students together. The purpose of such "togetherness" is to introduce students to the fact that after graduation they will be faced with the team approach in their professional life. This team approach is particularly difficult for physicians who have traditionally given orders which others followed. In these situations a number of questions arise such as: "Whose diagnostic acumen is most respected?" or "Who initiates treatment?" "Who prescribes medication?" These issues are of course the outcome of the new role of nurse-practitioners.[40]

In addition to using the team approach to cut costs, hospitals, and particularly those owned and operated by health maintenance organizations, rush patients through so-called "accelerated care." The purpose of this approach is to increase the profits of HMOs to the maximum even as patients are moved from suture to discharge in less than 48 hours. This high speed "treatment" is achieved by having nurses draw blood, do an EKG or electrocardiograph and also teach patients about medication. All of these tasks were at one time done by specialists. In the mad rush to move patients in and out of the hospitals, baths, backrubs and any kind of personal attention to the patients is gone. Some have called this "hit and run" nursing. In California, 7,500 members of the California Nurses Association went on strike against Kaiser Permanente hospitals in 1997 until that HMO agreed to let the union select an 18 member nurse quality committee. This was prompted by deaths in Kaiser hospitals caused by inattention and the use of low-skilled workers as well as the stress put on nurses whose ranks had been sharply reduced in layoffs.[41]

The future of nursing in America has already been determined. That future is the permanent addition of the nurse-practitioner to the health delivery system in the United States. Indeed, the profit motive on the part of health maintenance organizations has led to the substitution of nurses for physicians as the primary care "doctors" in many communities. In part, this development was the result of the great anxiety of physicians to specialize and earn larger and larger fees. As the costs of health care increased, employers kept pressuring health maintenance organizations to keep the premiums down. This in turn led to the present state of health care in America in which a glut of specialists and a dearth of primary care physicians unintentionally "invited" the up-grading of nurses to the nurse-practitioner role. Nurse practitioners seldom earn more than $65,000 a year in sharp contrast to primary care physicians who average $135 thousand per year.[42]

It can be assumed that nursing will continue to be professionalized. The best indication for this assumption is the establishment of the National Center for Nursing Research. This indicates that the profession has recognized that research is the basis for professional progress in any field of human endeavor because that which does not progress, dies. The National Center for Nursing Research focuses on both acute and potential health problems. This is done by attempting to prevent disease and by promoting health. For example, the profession has been active in trying to reduce smoking, particularly among children even as the profession has encouraged numerous preventive measures such as exercise, nutrition and public health measures.

One of the consequences of the increased status nurses have attained for themselves by usurping the doctor's "turf" is that the same shift in professional responsibility which has benefitted the nursing profession now threatens to undermine their authority. Financial considerations have led to the introduction of so called "ancillary" personnel into hospitals and doctor's offices. These ancillaries label their tasks "nursing" and thereby threaten to take away at one end what has been gained by the profession at the other end.[43]

Nurses, like all American professionals, will be faced with two major changes in their ranks. These changes concern gender equality and racial and cultural diversity. At present, only 4 percent of American nurses are black. Those blacks who are in nursing blame this situation on racism while white nurses usually claim that blacks have poorer preparation and lower grades in high school and college than whites. They believe that blacks are generally not educationally motivated to gain jobs in areas depending on a high degree of education and skill. Whatever the reason for the under representation of blacks in the nursing profession, black nurses founded the National Black Nurses Association in 1971 "for the professional development of the professional black nurse."[44]

Because more black nursing students are enrolled in associate degree programs than in any other type, the NBNA claims that this enrollment is the product of racism. Because black nursing students seldom engage in study leading to the B.N.S. degree it is certain that leading positions in the profession will seldom be allocated to a black. Racism, combined with this apparent lack of education, will continue to lead to a dearth of blacks in administrative and teaching positions in nursing.[45]

Men are also grossly under-represented in nursing. The reasons for this imbalance lie mainly in popular conceptions of the male role in American life. Thus, many Americans believe that men who enter nursing must be homosexuals. Further, it is commonly believed that men who enter "female" occupations do not make good role models for their children. In addition it is believed that men who enter nursing must have failed at more masculine professions such as medicine, dentistry or pharmacy. These beliefs are contradicted by male nursing students and male nurses. Thus, Anders reports that his own survey showed that men who enter nursing are primarily motivated to enter nursing because they "liked people and enjoyed helping others." Job availability and job security were also cited by male nurses as reasons for entering the profession. Others said that they had a great deal of interest in the biological sciences. Most male nurses seek to enter traditional male settings such as emergency rooms, intensive care units and anesthesia units in their nursing career.[46]

Male nursing students are generally older than female nursing students because many of them had failed at another occupation before entering nursing school. This fact may bear out one of the popular beliefs about male nurses. Men in the nursing profession must also be re-socialized. This means that men in the profession must at least understand the female point of view or act in a manner reflecting female attitudes and roles. Since men are not usually attuned to occupations involving the care of other people, men must first learn the care-giver role, a role women have already accepted at a younger age. Male nurses also have to learn to examine women, an activity few men have ever learned and one that their patients seldom expect. A male nurse must also learn how to get along with a mainly female nursing staff.

Teamwork is very important in nursing. Therefore male nurses have to learn to work on a team with large numbers of women. Since the experiences of men and women differ, men have a different attitude than women have. Men in all walks of life have been taught that team work is very important. It is also probable that men have worked in situations other than nursing which require team work because team work is part of the American culture.[47]

Men who enter nursing must also learn to live with a great deal of criticism and discrimination. This criticism is related to the general American belief that male nurses are playing a female role and that nursing is a low prestige occupation. The fact is that nursing has held a middle range position in the prestige ratings of occupations in the Untied States for many years. Physicians have held the first rank among occupations in the opinion of Americans as long as such public opinion polls have been taken. Yet, pharmacists, veterinarians, teachers other than professors, accountants and librarians all rank lower than registered nurses in such prestige scales.[48]

Men in nursing reflect the same anxieties associated with any minority status. Gender role conflict is only one reason for such anxieties. Since sex role socialization begins at birth men in nursing will undoubtedly have to make some major adjustments when facing an overwhelmingly female world each day. It is of course true that the gender revolution which has permitted women to enter into many traditional male occupations has also furnished men with cause to enter nursing. Theoretically, then, men should have social permission to play a compassionate or caring role just as women now insist that they have the right to be assertive. Nevertheless, sexism is still a strong force in American culture so that men in nursing must continue to live with the rejection their career choice inevitably produces. It is of course possible that men in nursing are already more tender minded than other men. It is also possible that men who chose nursing because they could not meet the demands of the male economic world acquired some learned female characteristics in order to carry out the demands of the profession. For example, a comparison between male engineers and male nurses found that relationship factors are much more important to male nurses than to male engineers. [49]

In any event, male nurses encounter negative attitudes not only from their friends, relatives and acquaintances but also from the health care environment. Nowhere is that more in evidence than in the obstetrical or midwife area. Male nurses are a visible minority in that situation although most physicians who practice in that field are men. Nevertheless, even nurse educators have perpetuated stereotypes which are detrimental to men entering the field of obstetrical nursing. These attitudes lead to a great deal of discouragement for men seeking to enter obstetrical nursing. In fact, the anxiety produced by nurse educators concerning men in obstetrical nursing will suffice to discourage most male nurses to enter that field. This anxiety is produced by the beliefs of many obstetrical patients that men are unacceptable as obstetrical nurses. In addition, participation of male nurses in such deliveries is usually deemed unacceptable to female nursing students and others. Yet, male doctors find no such opposition to their participation in the birthing process.[50]

A study of 506 boys in a Rhode Island High School concluded that High School seniors view nursing as the least acceptable occupation for men. These students thought that the nursing occupation violates sex roles in vocational choice. Male high school seniors in that Rhode Island study agreed that male nurses are lazy and of low intelligence. There is, of course, no evidence that men in nursing are less intelligent than other men. It suffices that this is commonly believed in order to discourage men who are considering nursing as a career.

Despite all of these obstacles the number of men who have entered the profession of nursing at the end of the twentieth century has grown. Therefore, a larger and larger number of male role models will permit other men to make the same choice. A gradual decline in cultural prejudice against male nurses will develop in the next few years. This will improve the prestige of the occupation, increase the income of those serving in that capacity and contribute to gender equality for all those who must earn their livelihood.[51]

The essential issue relative to the earning of one's livelihood under optimum conditions is the need for power. The entire history of nursing so far has been the history of a powerless community dependent on the good will of doctors. Most recently, however, nurses have demanded and gotten some power to make their own decisions. In addition it is to be hoped that nursing education will cease to socialize nurses into sub-ordination. Nurses have recently succeeded in forming their own political action committee. Called Nurses Coalition for Action in Politics. This group seeks to resocialize women to gain equality with physicians and to conduct themselves as equals in the presence of physicians. It is of course argued by some that women in power create a good deal of hostility from men with less power and that therefore nurse executives are fired at increasing rates. Much of the hostility to nurses is derived from the fear of physicians who suspect that nurses are an economic threat to them. Hence, it is risky for nurses or women anywhere to be assertive. Nurses are therefore now attempting to reorganize hospitals from the present patriarchal structure to one in which equality of gender is taken for granted. Nurses believe that physicians now take credit for work and expertise delivered by nurses. Nurses also say that hospital administrators want nurses to do more and more without having authority to make their own decisions. Nurses hope to achieve professional equality by the use of political activism. Nurses' strikes and demands for better pay and better working conditions in many American towns and cities have underscored these demands.[52]

Summary

There are nearly two million registered nurses in the United States earning an average salary of $36,000 per year. There are also 600,000 licensed practical nurses earning about $25,000 per year. Presently the drive to save money is leading some legislatures to consider revoking state licensures. The same motive has led Medicare to reimburse nurse-practitioners instead of doctors. The federal government now has five programs subsidizing health care. All this had led to a stratified health delivery system ranging from utterly untrained to highly specialized physicians. As hospitals have "downsized" and laid off registered nurses, home-health care nursing has increased as has an interest in attaining nurse-practitioners licenses through further university based education.

Nurses are now functioning on their own and outside of institutions. They are responsible for the dying, for the old and for the very young even as so called "multiskilled" are used to cut costs in hospitals. Nursing is even now mainly the work of white women as a number of factors tend to limit the participation of minorities and men in the profession. Nurses say that their next objective must be the attainment of political power so that they can achieve equality with doctors.

Notes

1.   Kalish, *op.cit.*, p. 371.

2.   Kalish, *op.cit., p. 371*

3.   Kalish, *op.cit.*, p. 371.

4.   Bureau of Labor Statistics, *op.cit.* ,March12, 1998 table #32505

5.   Lucille A. Joel, "Your License to Practice," American Journal of Nursing, Vol.95, No. 11, November 1995, p. 7.

6.   Ivan Oransky and Jay Varma, "Nonphysicians Clinicians and the Future of Medicine," *JAMA*, Vol.277, No. 13, April 2, 1007, p. 1090.

7.   Connie Helmlinger, "ANA Hails Landmark Law as Nursing Victory," *AJN* Vol. 97, No. 10, October 1997, p. 16.

8.   Ruth R. Anderson and Reuben A. McDaniel, Jr., "Intensity of Registered Nurse Participation in Nursing Home Decision Making," *The Gerontologist,* Vol.38, No.1, February 1998, pp. 90-100.

9.   David Keepnews, "New Opportunities and Challenges for APRNs." *AJN* Vol. 98, No.1, January 1998, pp. 46-52.

10.   Max Weber, *The Protestant Ethic and the Spirit of Capitalism,* Talcott Parsons, Trans., New York, Scribner, 1956, p.24.

11.   Peter I. Buerhaus and Douglas O. Staiger, "Future of the Nurse Labor Market According to Executives in High-Managed Care Areas of the United States," *Image: Journal of Nursing Scholarship,* Vol. 29, No. 4, Fourth Quarter, 1997, pp. 313-318.

12.   American Association of Colleges of Nursing, "Baccalaureate nursing education for the future: Defining the essential elements," Washington, D.C., 1997.

13.   Patrick H. DeLeon, Diane K. Kjervik, Alan G. Kraut and Gary R. Vanden Bos, "Psychology and Nursing: A Natural Alliance, *American Psychologist,* Vol.40, No. 11, November 1985, p. 1153.

14.   Virginia Kenyon, *et al*, "Clinical competencies for community health nurses," *Public Health Nursing,* Vol. 7, No. 1, 1990, pp. 33-39.

15.   Katherine A. Meyer, "An Educational Program to Prepare Acute Care Nurses for a Transition to Home Health Care Nursing," *The Journal of Continuing Education in Nursing,* Vol.28, No. 3, May/June 1987, pp,124-129.

16.   Nancy Shute, "A surge in graduate programs for nurses," *U.S. News and World Report,* March 2, 1998, p. 89.

17.   Associated Press, "Syracuse nursing students seek lawyer in administrative mix-up," The Buffalo News, August 11, 1998, p. A-4.

18.   Janet Cromley, "When Your Doctor is a Nurse," *Good Housekeeping,* " Vol. 225, No.2, August 1997, pp. 145-146.

19.   Lorraine Aiken, "Transformation of the nursing workforce," *Nursing Outlook,* Vol.43, No.5, 1995, pp. 201-209.

20.   Larry Dossey, *Space, Time & Medicine,* New Science Library, Boston, 1982.

21.   Deborah Witt Sherman, "Correlates of Death Anxiety in Nurses Who Provide AIDS Care," *Omega,* Vol. 34, No.2, 1996-1997, pp. 117-136.

22.   Cheryl Tatano Beck, "Nursing Students' Experiences Caring for Dying Patients," *Journal of Nursing Education,* Vol. 36, No.9, November 1997, pp. 408-415.

23.   Art Moore, "Hospice Care Hijacked," *Christianity Today,* Vol.42, No.3, March 2, 1998, pp. 38-41. .

24.   *Ibid.* p. 39.

25.   H.E.Stuck and H,U. Aronow, "A trial of annual in-home comprehensive geriatric assessments for elderly people living in the community," *New England Journal of Medicine,* Vol. 333, No. 18, 1995, p. 1184.

26.   Carole Kelly, "Surveyeing Public Health Nurses' Continuing Education Needs: Collaboration of Practice and Academia," *The Journal of Continuing Education in Nursing,* Vol. 25, No3, May-June 1997, pp. 115-123.

27.   Lauren Hunter and Vanda Lops, "Certified Nurse Midwives," JAMA, Vol. 277, No.13, April 2, 1997, p. 1095.

28.   Susan Brown and Dorothy Grimes, "Who's number one in primary care, RNs or MDs ?" *RN,* Vol.59, No. 4, April, 1996, p. 16

29.   Elaine Brainerd, "School Health Nursing Services Profess Review: Report of 1996 National Meeting," *Journal of School Health,* Vol. 68, No.1, January 1998, p.12.

30.   Carole A. Anderson, "Nurses to Recommend Provider Mix in Shortage Areas," *Public Health Reports,* Vol. 113, No. 1, January/February 1998, p. 113.

31.   Jean Nagelkerk, Patricia M. Ritola and Patty J. Vandort, "Nursing Informatics: The Trend of the Future," *The Journal of Continuing Education in Nursing,* Vol.29, No. 1, January/February 1998, p. 17.

32.   Lynette Leeseberg Stamler and Barbara Thomas, "Patient Stories: A Way to Enhance Continuing Education," *Journal of Continuing Education in Nursing,* Vol. 28, No. 2, March/April 1997, pp. 64-68.

33.   Stanley J. Heymann, "Patients in Research: Not just subjects, but partners." *Science,* Vol. 269, pp. 797-798.

34.   Sally Thomas and Gale Hume, "Delegation Competencies: Beginning Practitioners' Reflections," *Nurse Educator,* Vol. 23, No. 1, January-February 1998, p. 38.

35.   Suzanne Gordon, "The Quality of Mercy," *The Atlantic Monthly,* Vol. 279, No. 2, February,1979 p.81.

36.   Gerhard Falk, *Sex, Gender and Social Change; The Great Revolution,* Lanham, MD., The University Press of America, 1998.

37.   Gordon, *op.cit.* p. 87.

38.   Barbara L. Paterson, "The Negotiated Order of Clinical Teaching," *Journal of Nursing Education,* Vol.36, No. 5, May 1997, pp. 197-205.

39.   *Ibid.* p. 205.

40.   Circe Cook, " Reflections on the Health Care Team: My Experiences in an Interdisciplinary Program." *JAMA,* Vol.277, No. 13, April 2, 1997, p. 1091.

41.   Peter T. Kilborn, "Nurses Get New Role in Patient Protection," *The New York Times,* March 26, 1998, p. A 14.

42.   Milt Freudenheim, "Nurses Treading on Doctor's Turf," *The New York Times,* Nov. 2, 1997, Sec. 4, p. 5.

43.   Janice B. Lindberg, Mary Love Hunter and Ann Z. Kruszewski, *Introduction to Nursing,* Philadelphia, Lipppincott-Raven Publishers, 1998, pp. 428-429.

44.   Jeanette Vaughan, "Is There Really Racism in Nursing?" Journal of Nursing Education, Vol. 36, No. 3, March 1997, pp. 135-139.

45.   Ibid. p. 137.

46.   Robert L. Anders, "Targeting Male Students," *Nurse Educator,* Vol. 18, No.2, March/April, 1993, p. 4.

47.   Helen J. Steubert, "Male Nursing Students' Perception of Clinical Experience," *Nurse Educator,* Vol. 19, No.5, September-October 1994, pp. 28-32.

48.   Beth B. Hess, Elizabeth W. Markson and Peter J. Stein, *Sociology,* New York, Macmillan Publishing Co., 1991, p. 179.

49.   Michael Galbraith, "Attracting Men to Nursing: What Will They Find Important in Their Career?" *Journal of Nursing Education,* Vol. 30, No.4, April 1991, pp. 182-186.

50.   Roy A. Sherrod, "The Role of the Nurse Educator: When the Obstetrical Nursing Student is Male," *Journal of Nursing Education,* Vol.28, No.8, October 1989, pp. 377-379.

51.   Shirley Davis-Martin, "Research on Males in Nursing," *Journal of Nursing Education,* Vol. 23, No. 4, April 1984, pp. 162-164.

52.   Joan J. Roberts and Thetis M. Group, *Feminism in Nursing,* Westport, Con. Praeger, 1995, pp. 330-331.

Chapter III
The Perpetrators

In every profession there are people who deviate from the norm. In the occupation of nursing this may come as a surprise because of the expected ethics in that field. It is especially noticed since the majority of nurses are caring trusted professionals.

The Perpetrators or Respondents, as they are known in the disciplinary sessions of a State Nurse Board are nurses who have wittingly or unwittingly committed unacceptable actions, behaviors toward patients, the welfare of others, their profession and the public. Their conduct may be harmful, fallacious or criminal. The following cases will here describe some of these nurses and the situations in which such acts occurred. The names of the nurses as well as the geographic areas in which the situations occurred are concealed to protect the identity of the persons in question. These cases describe real people who appeared before a court, or a panel of a three to five member "jury" of a nurse board for examination and determination of guilt.

Nurse Louise Maxine a very attractive LPN was employed by a hospital in a mid western city. She was well liked by fellow staff members and was friendly and outwardly accommodating to the patients on her floor. One of the patients under her care became very ill, had difficulty breathing and began to lose consciousness. Nurse Maxine telephoned the resident doctor describing the state of her very ill patient and was asking him to come at once to see him. Before the physician appeared the patient, Mr. Keehan, died. This occurred in a matter of minutes from the time that the telephone call was made until the doctor arrived. Great concern was exhibited by Nurse Maxine and she was praised by the staff and the Doctor for attempting to help the patient. Several other patients on Ms. Maxine's shift had died in previous months and were assisted by the Nurse in an attempt to revive them. They all had exhibited the same symptoms and no reason was found for the sudden death of these people. She had tried to rescue them from their fate and always searched out an M.D. to assist in the last few seconds of the lives of these folks. Mr. Keehan's sudden death was unexpected since he was a patient who seemed to have been getting along well prior to the final episode. It such a shock to his sons that they insisted on a post mortem examination. It was found that he had an excessive amount of insulin in his body in spite of the fact that he was not a severe diabetic. Nurse M. had injected him with a massive dosage of the drug, had wanted to show what a rescuer she is, wanted recognition for her deed but failed to bring him "back" to life.

Upon closer investigation it was learned that Ms. Maxine had a long history of dysfunctional behavior. She was doing some gratis home care for her uncle when she decided to ignite his bed while he was sleeping. She was "fed up doing gratis work." Fortunately he woke up in time to smell the smoke and to see the flames emanating from beneath his mattress. He was able to roll out of bed and escape the tragedy of being burned alive. His nurse niece seeing him alive denied any part in having been involved in this fiery episode. It was shortly thereafter that the Uncle moved into a nursing facility.

Ultimately this nurse was convicted of the death of Mr. Keehan. Although this was not the only murder that she had perpetrated, it was the only one that could be proven for which she was responsible and for which she was incarcerated. She was sentenced to fifteen years in a maximum security prison.

Junta Josina is a pleasant appearing, impeccably dressed black registered nurse with a delightful Caribbean accent. She came to the United States having received her training in her native island. She had been employed in the obstetrics/gynecology department of a large metropolitan hospital. She smiled in a charming fashion, nodding a greeting to each member of the nurse board jury as well as to the prosecutor, administrator, and court reporter who were gathered in the room.

This nurse was brought before the Disciplinary Board because of a situation in which she was the primary care giver and nurse of a young female patient. Junta Josina was the night nurse who had been assigned to this case and who was responsible for her care and well being. A very pregnant woman arrived late one evening in the emergency room since she was experiencing strong labor pains. Shortly after her arrival she was taken to the obstetrics floor and from there to the labor suite. Junta was the nurse in charge and she noticed that Rose was having contractions every few minutes. Nurse Josina waited patiently until the woman's contractions were two minutes apart before she listened to the patient's abdomen with a stethoscope. Rose was in severe distress, screaming in pain. Nurse Josina did not show a great deal of concern since she had heard the cries of women who were in labor almost on a daily basis. She covered her ears with both hands because she was very much annoyed about the "carryings on" of this aching and unhappy patient. After hours of struggling and expressions of severe pain, patient Rose was sweating and exhausted. She became very still and looked asleep although her eyes were open. Junta was under the erroneous impression that the situation was under control and believed that all was within normal limits and did not call in the resident obstetrician to examine the patient. (She was always hesitant to awaken the doctors and was intimidated by them.) Nurse Josina was relieved because she did not have to hear the woman's screams and could resume reading her True Romance book. When the supervising nurse appeared to make the rounds of the ward she tried to listened to the infant's heart beat and that of the mother. She heard nothing.

Months later Nurse Josina was called to the nurse board hearing where she was confronted with the neglect and pain that had been suffered by her erstwhile patient. She was asked whether she listened to the abdomen with a fetal monitor. Junta could not imagine what was meant by the word "fetal monitor" until she understood that it was the stethoscope that was utilized to listen for heart sounds. She was asked what she heard when going over the examination of the woman's abdomen. She confessed that she heard no heart beat and believed that "the unborn baby was sleeping." Although the members of the jury panel were very dejected over the outcome of this case they could not help laughing at the ignorance of Nurse Josina, and that this registered nurse did not know nor comprehend that awake or asleep the human heart keeps beating until life ceases. Nurse Josina was surprised when she learned that the baby had died within the mother's womb and that the mother had suffered severe brain damage. Needless to say Junta was ignorant about nursing procedures, physiology and the duties and tasks that her position as an alleged registered graduate nurse entailed. It goes without saying that Nurse Josina lost her nursing license as well as having a serious penalty placed upon her. This respondent felt that she was severely psychologically injured and believed herself to have suffered from discriminatory practices and totally unfair treatment when the questioning of the nurse board members persisted and ultimately when her fate was sealed and the verdict to remove her license was made.

Susan Grimsby a handsome looking tall woman impeccably groomed and suited with a conspicuously large cross adorning her tailored suit smiled broadly at "the audience" as she entered the assembled jury room. Her demeanor was one of self assurance, confidence and controlled possession of her emotions. She made an effort to engage the members of the panel in conversation and hoped to encounter their good will in dealing with the situation at hand. Susan was a graduate of a hospital nursing school, had continued at the local university for her bachelors degree and was in preparation for her Masters degree at the same university. Her credentials looked impressive as did her outer appearance. For the past several years Susan had become the Director of Nursing in a small Catholic nursing facility for nuns. She had several registered nurses working under her direction as well as a number of aides and other staff and personnel. The third floor of this facility held the most frail elderly nun patients, many of them between the ages of eighty two and one hundred. Some were not as coherent or expressive as one would like but others were alert and bright. These patients had served the young, the old, the poor and the vulnerable They had been educators, nurses and care givers most of their lives and now in their current state could expect to live a tranquil and as comfortable a life as their spiritual, physical and emotional state would permit. The majority were very docile women who readily accepted with gratitude any help and assistance given them in their waning years that were left them. Their faith and spirituality carried them through the vagaries of illness and disability that they were facing in their last stage on earth.

These very gentle and aged women had earned the right to be treated with kindness, compassion and respect. They had earned this throughout their years of serving the most wanting and needy of humanity, had given of themselves without monetary rewards and had done so willingly and generously without remorse. This was not the belief or conviction of Nurse Grimsby. She was determined to oversee her patients in a controlling fashion and to dictate to them and to their keepers what and how they were to eat, to sleep, to dress and to conduct themselves. She had a harsh domineering way of speaking about and with them and attempted to coerce them to follow her dictates. In addition she had her favorites among the staff and would imbue her "ways" unto them, would allow them more freedom if they agreed with her. One aide was her very favorite and this woman would carry out the orders of nurse Susan to the minutest detail. The remainder of the employees were ordered about in an often irrational manner and were given the most undesirable tasks and working hours imaginable. Her pet aide was protected from all that and chose whatever she wanted concerning her work times and duties. Susan and Aide Carey seemed to be closely connected to one another. This situation created poor morale and unhappy feelings among the caregivers of the institution. Although Nurse Grimsby professed to love the "little old" nuns who were in her care she viewed them with disdain and derision and was frequently heard laughing at them for being who they were.

We must look at the background of Ms. Grimsby to understand her thoughts and actions in her dealings with "her" patients and "her staff." She was the product of the Catholic Schools and revealed that she was abused by her nun teachers whom she despised. She was determined to "get even" with them but could do nothing about it as she was growing up. She made up for her then helplessness by punishing the frail nuns whom Nurse Susan was now able to control. She not only detested these women but was an ageist in addition to her specific hatreds around her religion and the mistreatment that she felt she had experienced as a child. She believed in the adage "an eye for an eye" even if the proverbial eyes that she eviscerated were those of innocent, helpless, vulnerable victims who had nothing to do with Susan's childhood experiences or misfortunes.

Susan was called before the disciplinary board of nursing because she had six specifications of professional misconduct as follows: She was charged with practicing the profession of nursing with gross negligence, with gross incompetence, with negligence on more than one occasion and with committing unprofessional behavior by physically and verbally abusing patients; by unlawfully delegating nursing duties and by committing conduct which evidences moral unfitness, while employed in the Sisters of Mercy Home and Infirmary and Convent in "Allentown, New York" as a registered professional nurse, Susan unlawfully delegated the duties of performing treatments and of administering medications to unlicensed personnel. She did not follow the nurse practice act. The Respondent was hired to perform treatments and to prepare and administer medications to the patients/ residents of the Infirmary Convent on her shift. The second specification of misconduct consisted of force feeding and willfully abusing senior citizen patients until they choked and vomited. One of the force fed nuns who was treated in this manner by Susan would weep and beg the RN to stop but the caregiver only laughed and ridiculed her. There is real cause to believe that a sister Lazimira died as the result of one of these episodes. She choked on the food which Susan virtually shoveled into her mouth. This very old nun was despised by the aforementioned RN and appeared to get sadistic pleasure from seeing this frail, tiny lady struggle for breath. She took no responsibility for this woman's ultimate death and was overheard by one of the staff exclaiming: "It's about time this old creep is leaving us." Other nuns who were able to feed themselves were force-fed at a very rapid speed which caused much coughing, choking and gastro intestinal distress. A witness testified regarding these allegations and a second staff member spoke to the authenticity and honesty of the witness.

Nurse Susan was also in the habit of screaming at the nuns. It is true that many of the patients were hard of hearing but the voice of Nurse Susan when she had "one of her shouting/screaming attacks" could be heard in the entire building. If a nun dropped a utensil or spilled a bit of liquid she would demand that she leave the dining room at once. She would threaten the patients that if they did not obey her they would end up in hell. She would also call them names like "fat pig," informed them that they had been abandoned by their families, that they were disliked and had completed their task in this world and should realize that it was overdue for them to die. Those patients who had to wear neck braces were at times gasping for breath since Nurse Susan had tightened them excessively creating severe discomfort for the sufferers. If a nun would not respond to Susan's demands to leave the dining room she would push, shove and drag the individual out. One nun, a Sister Rosalinda was slapped by the RN who tore her habit in a fit of anger. Rosalinda wept uncontrollably following this incident. One nun who had difficulty swallowing was fed with a syringe. When she vomited RN Susan fed the nun the vomit "to teach her a lesson for spitting out food."

Although the administrator of the facility was a registered nurse herself as well as a nun, she refused to believe the staff who hesitantly came to report Susan's misdeeds. She felt that the reporters disliked Susan for various reasons and no longer wanted her "excellent and necessary supervision;" that they were rightfully chastised by Susan; that she, the administrator, did not want to overstep her bounds; that she was very naïve and trusting and additionally had been flattered by the aforementioned supervisor and been impressed by her theoretical knowledge of nursing procedures. Thus Susan had the opportunity to practice her mephistophelean deeds for an extended period of time. It took a great deal of courage on the part of the staff members and often a loss of their jobs to be persistent in their reports to succeed in pressuring the Administrator to personally investigate the allegations.

There were enough witnesses in the case of Susan that there was no doubt of the authenticity that this very hostile, sadistic nurse was extremely abusive to the fragile, vulnerable elderly patients that were in her "care." Many witnesses were called to testify in this situation and several years passed before the case was concluded. Susan had an attorney who attempted to bring evidence that the respondent's witnesses were biased against her for personal vendettas. It took a great deal of investigation and effort to verify and authenticate the charges brought against this character disordered woman. She exhibited a lack of conscience and no remorse for the brutalities that she perpetrated. It was with one voice that all members of the jury unanimously agreed upon the final decision: This erstwhile nurse lost her license to practice the profession of nursing. It is unfortunate for the public that such an individual can ultimately get a position where she can conceivably do more harm in the future.

Boris Korlios was an experienced RN. in his forty second year of life he worked in a large urban hospital. He was friendly to patients and well respected by other staff members. He worked the evening shift and preferred that schedule because it was convenient for him. It gave him an opportunity to work on his bachelor's degree and freed the morning for that purpose. He declared that he had no interest in going out at night and stated that he missed nothing as a result of his shift. One evening he was working with a sixteen year old male patient, Michael, who had recently fractured his leg and hip. The patient screamed out for help. His injuries were the result of a fall from a motorcycle accident. His screams were heard by several aides coming from the direction of this boys room. They together investigated the situation when they saw Boris scurry out of the room in great haste. Boris explained that the boy is in severe pain and he, Boris, is taking care of the boy. He urged the two people to go back to their tasks and to leave his patient for him. There was allegedly nothing to be concerned about according to this RN Later when the one aide peered into Michael's room he found him weeping uncontrollably and begging to be permitted to call his mother. He was extremely distressed, red faced and sobbing. When the RN had busied himself with another case the aide found a portable phone and gave it to the young man to use. Amidst sobs he was overheard telling his parent that he had been sexually molested by Boris and he wanted his mother to come to the hospital at once. The mother came within the hour and found the head nurse working on the same floor where her son's room was located in order to report what had happened to her boy. As a result of this allegation of molestation, Boris was summoned by the administration and confronted. He categorically denied the charge with great vehemence. He claimed that he had merely given Michael the "usual and necessary care" which had been misinterpreted by the sixteen year old. Michael was questioned in detail and it was determined that he had indeed been molested by his care giver. With great shame and embarrassment he told how Boris had masturbated him against his will and had performed oral sex on him. His repulsion of this uninvited homosexual "rape" was so great that Michael was seen by a psychiatrist and his allegations were validated. Michael had been violated and was suffering from the trauma that was such a shock to him. Boris was discharged from his position, ultimately had to appear before the disciplinary jury of the Nurse Board. His license was revoked, a fine was invoked as well and compulsory psychiatric treatment instituted. Boris was barred from his profession for the foreseeable future.

James Crasso, a licensed registered nurse was employed in the emergency room of a mid sized urban hospital. He had worked in that position for five years and appeared to have been a "good, conscientious employee" according to his peers and supervisors. His appearance was that of a muscular strong looking male who was able to lift and transfer patients with skill and ease. He was always willing to assist with tasks that were difficult for the less muscular nurses to handle.

Because of this nurse's reputation it came as a shock to his cohorts when he was accused of molesting a male patient while he was at work on the evening shift in the emergency room. Patient Rex was admitted that night on a stretcher in restraints after a very volatile situation had occurred. The next morning while speaking to his psychiatrist this patient reported that he had been molested by the nurse in attendance, Mr. James Crasso. The patient had described in detail that the nurse had let him out of his restraints, took him to the bathroom because he had difficulty urinating and rubbed Vaseline all over his penis. The episode was reported to the Director of Nursing and she, together with the union representative, Crasso's supervisor and RN Crasso met to discuss the situation. The nurse in his own defense stated that he attempted to obtain a urine specimen from the patient while the patient was restrained on a stretcher. In order to do so, he had to place the patient's penis in a urinal, although the patient was not able to urinate. Nurse Crasso further stated at that meeting, that when the patient later said he had to urinate, the Nurse had a security guard release the patient from his restraints and took him to the toilet. With the security guard posted outside the door to the bathroom, Nurse Crasso stated that he ran the water but the patient was still unable to urinate. The nurse claimed that he escorted the patient back to his stretcher. In a written statement prepared by the Nurse, he reiterated the above attempts to obtain a urine specimen and noted that, as they were leaving the bathroom, he told Patient Rex: "Now don't say anything," to which the patient replied, "Okay." Nurse Crasso further wrote that this was a sort of warning to the patient that, if he remained calm, perhaps one hand might be left unrestrained.

Several days later and in light of Mr. Crasso's denial, together with the Patient's alcohol level and psychiatric history, the Director of Nursing concluded that the patient's allegations that respondent had rubbed lotion on his penis were unsubstantiated.

Five months thereafter a patient, James K., was admitted to the Hospital's emergency room for treatment of renal failure. He told his nurse that he had sought treatment for the same problem on several occasions at another facility. He had experienced a prior unfortunate incident with a male nurse and he feared being treated again by the same nurse, whom he had seen on duty that evening. After some encouragement this patient reported to his nurse that, some months ago a male nurse, whom the patient described, followed him into the bathroom and offered to assist him in obtaining a urine specimen. He further reported that he became alarmed and could not urinate, at which time the nurse "grabbed" his penis and began to vigorously massage it. The patient told the nurse to let him go, that he did not need help and the patient left the bathroom. The Director of Nursing was notified of this patient's allegations. The nurse in question, Mr. Crasso was notified and he in turn called on his Union representative for assistance once more.

A short time later the union representative, the director of nursing, Mr. Crasso and his immediate supervisor met and discussed the situation in question. Nurse Crasso insisted that he did rub a patient's penis with surgilube to help him urinate, but there was no sexual meaning to this. He insisted that he had only done this on one or two occasions and it was possible that patient James was one of them. Crasso further declared that he had put the lubricant on his hand solely for stimulating urination with the help of the aforementioned massage. He conceded that patient James might have been one of the patient's who needed his help, although this Patients's face was familiar, he did not recall the details of that patient's treatment.

Nurse Crasso was asked why he thought it would be appropriate to massage a patient's penis with surgilube on his hand, he responded that he had learned this very helpful technique while he was a nurse at another teaching facility.

Nurse Crasso later changed his story and alleged that he had squeezed the lubricant on the hand of the patient so that this man could massage his own penis.

When the case of Crasso came before the jury panel of the Nurse Board, for the second time. Nurse Crasso denied any previous statements made and was adamant in testifying that he never massaged any patient's penis and that he never made such a statement previously. Nurse Crasso had brought with him as witness, his union representative, who agreed with the Nurse denying any statements that had allegedly been made on previous occasions. A number of witnesses were called who had been at the previous meetings and all very strongly insisted that Nurse Crasso had in previous sessions told them that he had massaged the penis of said patient.

There were three separate sessions before the nurse board panel of five jurors, witnesses and attorneys for both the defendant and the Nurse Board. There was much deliberation. After denial and counter denial and contradictions on the part of Mr. Crasso, the jury panel rejected as not credible the testimony of Nurse C. and that of the union representative that he had not massaged patient James penis. The panel further rejected as incredible the Nurse's testimony that he never massaged any person's penis. The jury unanimously agreed that the respondent James had escorted Patient James to the bathroom where the respondent applied surgilube to his hand and massaged the patient's penis. The respondent performed said act without a physician's order, medical justification or necessity but rather, for his own gratification. This act occurred on more than on one occasion.

Determination as to guilt: It was unanimously determined that the charges contained in the above specifications have been proven by a preponderance of the evidence and that the respondent is guilty of the same. The penalty that was imposed unanimously by the jury panel of the Nurse Board was: Revocation of the respondent's license to practice as a registered professional nurse in the State. It should here be noted that this man cannot practice as an RN in any state since the revocation will appear electronically if ever he decides to apply for a license anywhere in this United States of America.

Ertha Kalonetta RN was employed in a City Hospital for two years. Her education came from a qualified hospital school of nursing and her grades while a student were acceptable. Prior to the City Hospital position she served as staff nurse in a number of other reputable institutions. There were no known sanctions in the records of her past employments and there was no reason to believe that she could not fulfill any job in her particular field. It was noted by her colleagues that she did not seem to follow the physicians orders and seemed to want to be in control of the patients care without input from others. Ertha is a middle aged woman who made a good impression when she was first introduced to her colleagues. After a few months it was noticed that she was argumentative and insistent upon her way of thinking, that she always needed to be right and in control.

One day while she worked the eight a.m. to eight p.m. shift (she ordinarily had a three day, twelve hour shift) she was taking care of a vulnerable post surgery male patient. His needs were carefully documented by the physician to be followed as written. Among other directives this patient was to be given eye medication in order to retain his vision as well as to have a nutrition line until there would be an order to discontinue it. Nurse K. took it upon herself to turn off the feeding tube without a physician's directive and furthermore she did not administer the prescribed eye drops. The eye medication had been removed from the night table and in addition the nutrition line was no longer dispensing any food. When the next shift came on at eight a.m. the morning nurse noticed that the patient was dehydrated. He was fairly unresponsive and when RN K. was later questioned she at first adamantly denied that she had ignored any order given; she later stated she was certain that the patient in question did not need the tube feeding and that the eye drops had been given at another time and she felt this was sufficient. Her actions were contrary to what the doctor had prescribed for this patient. In addition she had not documented properly into the record what had transpired during her shift in relationship to this patient. The facts were that she had practiced nursing in a very negligent fashion. She had dozed during a portion of her shift and was irresponsible in carrying out the essentials of care for this ill, post surgery patient. It was found that she had lied about medications and that she had not given prescribed medications to patients at other times. She had documented a number of untruths in the medical records of other patients and at other times had not documented at all. Nurse K. also during the shift when she was responsible for the Patient, nurse Kaloneta failed to notice that said patient's I.V. (intravenous) site was reddened and/or she had failed to take appropriate action with the afore said condition.

When the nurse was questioned by her supervisors and eventually by members of the nurse board panel she alleged that her employers accused her of wrong doing because of her race. She tried to prove her case not only by denial but by questioning how many RN's were employed at City Hospital. Witness after witness both Afro-American and Caucasian regarding this case were brought before the nursing panel and all of them were first hand observers, peers and supervisors of the allegations that had been brought before the Nurse Board.

It was the decision of the jury to charge the nurse with negligence and unprofessional conduct and to take disciplinary action accordingly.

Elizabeth Royal did not resemble the meticulous, neat professional looking nurse that one would imagine as a stereotypical registered nurse. She is a rotund, somewhat untidy appearing person with an abbreviated straight haircut, short in stature with a grim facial expression. She chose to be a "prison nurse" as a career. One could ponder whether she stepped into this role because she was unable to find other employment. Did she travel this path because the State's salaries were a bit higher than others, or did she feel she would not have to work as hard or have the work pressures that other nurses face? Did she possibly feel that "anything goes" because after all her patients are prisoners and their complaints would not be taken at face value, or were all of these issues the reason Nurse Royal found herself serving as a prison nurse?

Could she have in the remotest believed that she could teach these men how to be better citizens or did she hate them because they were in prison? These are all conjectures if we view the background and behaviors of this forty year old woman. When interviewed by this writer why she went into the practice of nursing she readily responded that she wanted to help people. Delving further into her background I learned that she had been abandoned by her mother when she was very young and that she was raised by a strict father who did not hesitate to use the rod. She seemed to have had very little affection in her life and always hoped that someone would accept her and love her. She was unable to find that for which she was searching. Not having been physically attractive nor having much feminine appeal she stated that she felt rejected most of her life. She had no illusion that the prisoners would find her any more appealing than anyone else would. Her obesity did not help her feelings of being unacceptable. She could release her anger and frustration unto the prisoners when she was in a bad mood or when they irritated her with their "ridiculous ailments." She would frequently ignore their requests for help or would become sarcastic toward them.

When she applied for jobs she frequently found herself rejected with some superficial excuses. She had held several other positions before the current one. In one of those beginning positions she felt exploited and left after a few months; in another job she felt the supervisor was "picking on" her, in a third she felt that the job was too strenuous for her and yet another she was informed that she would be better off if she found some other employment. In that job she resigned before she was terminated. It was at this juncture in her life at age thirty five that she decided to apply to a male prison to which a very small separate female addition was attached. The inmates ranged from men who had committed serious offenses to others who were incarcerated for less serious crimes. All, of course were in a "tightly locked" facility. She did as little as possible for the offenders and always went into the various cells with a prison guard. Although none of the guards were enamored with Elizabeth, she ascertained that she treated them with care lest they "turn on her" (as she explained it). She knew that if she did not adhere to the wishes of the guards they would let Nurse Elizabeth fend for herself. (There is always the risk in a prison that if the prison keepers/guards wanted they could expose other staff members to seriously dangerous acts). Such a fate RN Elizabeth did not want to test.

It was during Elizabeth's (now known as Respondent) employment at Incarcer prison that she was called before a disciplinary hearing of the State Board of Nursing for professional misconduct. At that time she was charged with ten specifications of professional misconduct which will be stated herewith:

1. The Respondent was charged with practicing the profession of nursing as a registered professional nurse with gross negligence, on a particular occasion within the purview and meaning of the State's Education Law. On or about July 4 to 5, 1998, Respondent was employed and on duty as a registered professional nurse on an overnight shift at said prison. Near the beginning of Respondent's shift on the evening of July 4, 1998, Respondent had been advised by the off-going nurse that inmate Gary Janus had a history of recent head trauma. Thereafter, Respondent failed to perform a nursing assessment of said inmate near the beginning of her shift; failed to monitor the inmate's condition as frequently as warranted; failed to thoroughly assess said inmate after Respondent became aware that he was unarousable; and failed to monitor said inmate after he became unarousable and was awaiting the arrival of an ambulance.

2. The Respondent was further charged with practicing the profession of nursing as a registered professional nurse with gross negligence on a particular occasion, within the purview and meaning of the State's Education Law in that: On or about July 16, 2000, while employed and on duty as a registered professional nurse at the Incarcer prison, Respondent failed to properly and thoroughly assess inmate Hank B. who had complaints of abdominal pain and of not having had a bowel movement for approximately three days prior thereto.

3. The Respondent was further charged with practicing the profession of nursing with gross negligence on a particular occasion, within the purview and meaning of the State's Education Law: On or about September 16 2000, Respondent was employed and on duty as an RN at the Incarcer Prison. After being informed by a licensed practical nurse that newly admitted inmate F. D. was an insulin dependent diabetic who took insulin twice a day, Respondent failed to assess said inmate, failed to ensure that a more thorough history was taken to determine when said inmate had last eaten and had last

taken insulin, and failed to ensure that a blood glucose test was promptly administered to said inmate.

4.   Respondent was further charged with practicing the profession of nursing as a registered professional nurse with gross negligence on a particular occasion, within the purview and meaning of the State's Education Law: In or about October 12, 2000, Respondent was employed and on duty as an RN at Incarcer Prison. On that date after a licensed practical nurse examined inmate N.X. because of a complaint of stomach pain, and after said licensed practical nurse requested Respondent to assess said inmate, Respondent failed for approximately two hours to assess said inmate who complained of stomach pain and recent vomiting, and failure to have a bowel movement for approximately one week prior thereto, and failed to request that said inmate be transferred to the infirmary or a hospital emergency room, when speaking with a physician about said inmate's care.

5.   Respondent was further charged with practicing the profession of nursing as an RN, with gross incompetence, within the purview of the State Education Law.

The allegations contained in the First Specification of professional misconduct are repeated, reiterated and re- alleged with the same force and effect as if more particularly set forth herein at length.

The sixth through tenth specifications of incompetence are all repeated for each of the above cases thus far stated.

Gary Janus, one of the first cases mentioned in this manuscript, had a history of recent head trauma and had refused treatment at a hospital before coming to the jail. He was examined on the evening shift by a nurse who treated his bleeding head wounds and who wanted to send him to the hospital. The respondent came on duty later that evening and received a report on Gary including his history of recent trauma. She failed to assess or even examine this patient during the first three hours of her shift. At about two o'clock in the morning when she heard jail personnel state that they could not wake the prisoner, an ambulance was ordered. The Respondent went to G's cell, looked at him lying on the floor. She gazed at him for approximately two seconds, then turned and walked out, leaving him unattended while awaiting an ambulance.

As to the second incident, the evidence showed that the Respondent saw the teenage inmate Hank B. during the early morning hours. Hank was complaining of abdominal pain and having been impacted without a bowel movement in three days. The Respondent performed the assessment of this prisoner through the bars from a distance; she remained outside the cell with the prisoner locked inside with severe pain. This was a non – assessment!

As the third incident the RN did not assess the prisoner, a woman, even though she had recently vomited and not moved her bowels for one week prior thereto. The inmate collapsed later that morning, was eventually transferred emergently to a hospital and died the next day of a hemorrhage due to a ruptured ectopic pregnancy.

By the preponderance of the evidence it was shown that Registered Nurse Elizabeth showed a shocking indifference to the well-being of the patients in her care. The jury in the case of this nurse decided to revoke this RN's license.

In an interview with Elizabeth the author obtained some insights into why this woman had chosen nursing as a profession and ultimately prison nursing. She was the oldest female child in a family of six children. The oldest offspring, John was a boy as were two of her younger siblings. Patrice, the girl a year Elizabeth's junior was a beautiful child, very much adored by her parents whereas Liz was ungainly, overweight and unattractive. Her parents were in poor economic circumstances, the father a day laborer, the mother cleaned houses to make a living. John was frequently left in charge of the younger children. He was an angry adolescent who enjoyed teasing and hurting the younger ones, especially Elizabeth whom he disliked. Thus she was frequently the object of his aggressions. He would pinch her, call her names and on a number of occasions he would force himself on her and sexually molest her.

Although she attempted to reveal this to her mother, this woman had no patience with the girl, and adding to her unhappiness, would not believe her and did not seem to be concerned or to care. The dad had no time for the children and especially not for this child. He would call her "fats" and would tell her to "stop feeding her ugly face." Elizabeth felt alienated from people and deserted by her parents; hatred from her brother; envious of the looks of Patrice and the love that was shown her sister. In addition she was burdened by the younger ones. The children in school ridiculed or ignored her altogether. As she grew older she was left out of the dating scene and often turned her anger on herself, becoming dejected and useless. Fortunately for Elizabeth she was a bright child and was able to achieve good marks in school. Since this brought her accolades from the teachers she expended a great deal of energy in pursuit of grades. She did succeed in that. She plotted in her mind to harm John and had day dreams about "getting even." She also had phantasies about being nurtured and cradled by a loving mother who cared only for her. Possibly unconsciously she believed that perhaps if she could cradle and love others she would feel good and would get love from her actions, becoming the loving parent that she never experienced. Thus as she graduated from high school she decided to become a nurse. She went about her studies with gusto and succeeded in receiving her much sought after diploma. Next came her search for a job. She had many interviews. She was sometimes rejected, sometimes not. One of the positions that was especially appealing to Liz was that of prison nurse. She experienced a feeling of exhilaration as she thought about the prisoners. She could even the score of those "evil" people who deserved to suffer. They would also have to tolerate her since she was the boss over these "low lives" who had probably raped women like herself and debased others. She also felt that the higher salary that was offered her for such a job would make up for the deprivations she had lived through as a child and young person. At the same time she feared these people who might injure her just as her brother John had. Should there be female prisoners she could show them who has the upper hand and who is needed. Thus Elizabeth chose the route of being a prison nurse.

When we examine this case with a critical eye we must wonder whether prison nurses are attracted by their ability to do as they please; that they don't care about people; that they want to punish prisoners who they feel have broken societies norms; that they are sadistic and enjoy their own hostilities or that they won't be detected nor does any one care how they treat the prisoners who are vulnerable people. Like a number of men and women who enter the occupation of prison guard they are not the most empathic or the kindest of individuals. The prison nurse is at the mercy and good will of the guards and if they dislike her she too becomes vulnerable and is in danger of being harmed by

> the more violent prisoners. She often sees things that are happening in the prison, unpalatable actions toward a prisoner that would under ordinary circumstances be contrary to the ethics of humane behavior and would call for reporting the perpetrator to the authorities. In a prison situation the nurse witnesses abuse of prisoners by guards and abuse by prisoners against one another. She fears the consequences of such observations on her part, thus she chooses to ignore that which she has learned from childhood and later from her knowledge of the teachings of morality and later from nursing ethics. To protect herself she chooses to either ignore the sadistic guards or worse still she joins them. Like the old adage: "If you can't lick them, join them."

The case of Roger Fortram is a very sad one. He was a young man who had a promising future. He was bright enough to be in the upper ten percent of the students of his high school class and had begun college when through some unfortunate circumstances he became entangled with a criminal gang and ultimately was involved in a serious crime which led to his incarceration in a maximum security prison. His youth had been a difficult one – he had been raised by a single Mom who because of her need to make a living was rarely at home. He never knew his Dad nor did he know anything about him. From the time he was very young he had to fend for himself and he had never felt the warmth of a caring environment. By the time Roger was twenty years of age he had reached his long term destination, namely Attran

Prison for serious felons. Somehow he did not fit in with the other prisoners in his compound. They were tough; they were hardened and for the most part considerably older than he. He was used by them for dubious purposes, ordered around by the other prisoners, manipulated and harshly treated by the staff. They addressed him by various unspeakable names including "Punk," manipulated him and belittled, embarrassed and abused him. There was not a day that passed by that he was not sexually assaulted by two or three older prisoners. Although the guards saw these abuses they did not interfere but seemed to gloat at the emotional and physical pain that he was suffering. By the time he had served one year in that devastating environment he began to act in a bizarre fashion. He screamed out quite often, would beat his head into his cell wall and would at times walk on all fours when let out into the "yard." One day after he had been drawn into a fracas between a group of inmates he was chosen to be locked into isolation. This was too much for him to bear. He screamed so loud, punched the bars in his cell and tapped his feet in a rhythmic fashion. The young man had broken from reality, he had become psychotic. One exceptionally large, strong guard unlocked the cell and dragged Roger out and kicked and beat him severely. Other guards added to this "amusement" and with Roger on the floor they kicked and beat him about the face and head. When the prisoner was seriously bleeding and had labored breathing they pulled him into the nurses "office" and told her "he's yours." She superficially examined him, did not notify the on call physician, nor an ambulance. She observed the man become unconscious and when he lay near death she merely shook her head and waited for him to die. Only then did Nurse Beatrice Blufton call an ambulance. He arrived at the community hospital dead! The nurse Blufton recorded this man's demise as: "Roger ceased to breathe, his respirations appeared to have stopped." The body was examined by a hospital physician and it became obvious that the death was caused as the result of the head and body blows that had been administered. The pathologist was without a doubt about the cause for the ultimate end of this young man's life.

It was not long following this situation that a distant relative of Roger saw the death notice of this erstwhile prisoner in the newspaper. She made some inquiries but was dissatisfied with the answers that were given. She duly notified the city's newspaper and an investigation began. One of the stories that occurred was: Prison Nurse let's Patient Die! The State's Nurse Board was notified and a disciplinary hearing was instituted!

Beatrice Blufton is a middle aged somewhat nondescript appearing woman who seemed fairly self assured to the uninitiated observer. She had been employed by the State Prison system for the past ten years. She had treated the prisoners in a matter of fact fashion but always seemed to have no sympathy for their pain or pleadings. She believed that they deserved the fate that led them to their position and she was unforgiving for their faults or what led them to their current dilemma. Her common response to physical pain was: "If you hadn't hurt others you wouldn't hurt now, so deal with it and stop whining." For psychological problems she had no use and would state that they had better change their behavior and "stop being crazy." She also made some pseudo religious pronouncements about "the Lord pays you back for what you did." Mercy did not exist in her vocabulary. She had nothing to fear when she dealt with an inmate since she was always surrounded by one or two guards when seeing one of the inmates. She made it her rule that she would never see more than one prisoner at any one time. She preferred that the person be in handcuffs if she needed to examine him. This of course was not always possible under the circumstances. She detested cleaning up body fluids and was known to have a sick prisoner clean up his own emissions, if and when an "accident" occurred. Gentle ministering and wound application was not one of the ways of Nurse Blufton.

When the pseudo conscious Roger was dragged along the floor toward Beatrice Blufton she was disgusted looking at this bleeding disheveled human. With rapid speed she donned her plastic gloves and demanded the guards place him on the cot which was standing near a wall of her small cubicle. After glancing at him with a repugnant look for some time she lifted his limp wrist and took his pulse. She then had the nearby guard open his tattered shirt while she stared at him for some time before placing a stethoscope to his chest. Having done that she busied herself wiping the stethoscope with alcohol while shaking her head in disgust. She and the two guards engaged in some damning conversation concerning the patient which contained such language as "that crazy bastard got what was coming to him." Much time passed before the dying Roger Fortram was loaded unto the gurney of the ambulance which took him for his final journey. No one in the prison seemed to care that this was once a living functioning human being; a baby, a child, an innocent creature who had a future. No one held his hand or gave him comfort as he left this world as a number, surrounded by cruel strangers.

It was many months later that Ms. Blufton appeared before the State Board of Nursing immaculately attired accompanied by her attorney. She was seated next to him behind a table facing a panel of six people which included four nurses, a public member (a private citizen) and an attorney for the State. The State's prosecutor was present in addition and the "trial," known as the disciplinary hearing began. Presentations were made about the many specifications of unprofessional and neglectful conduct on the part of the registered nurse, which ultimately led to the wrongful death of the prisoner/patient. Witnesses were called in behalf and against the actions of the nurse. There was an "expert" witness called, a Dean of a Nursing school who explained professional conduct and what is considered good and poor practice for one in the nursing field. There were individuals who knew the Nurse on a personal level and staff who knew her from the prison. Each reported what they felt and what was witnessed. There was much discussion and counter discussion. The nurse herself stated her case. She was exceptionally skillful in attempting to remove any responsibility for the outcome of the situation which brought her to the hearing. Her demeanor was one of defensiveness. In spite of her superficial smile the coldness that she exuded was unmistakable and filled the room with an ominous sense of dread.

She made every effort to mask her part in the problem by telling the panel of the dangers that lurk in prison and how careful one has to be when dealing with incarcerated felons. If one listened long enough the Nurse made it appear that she, not the Deceased was the victimized one. She let it be known if one were not in agreement with the prison guards and did not get along with them or joined in with their behaviors and cruelties the "poor prison nurse" would be vulnerable and would be left to her own devices to perish in prison at the hands of these "violent criminals." She even managed to squeeze out a few tears in an attempt to be convincing of her stance of total innocence, of herself as the victimized one.

Blufton's attorney made a lengthy statement about the RN's past, her loyalty, her longevity on the job; how she had always wanted to be a nurse, how much her nursing career and license meant to her, how much work and struggle she invested in her education, how she allegedly was always a "very caring" individual. He spoke about her "wonderful" parents who needed her. He brought forth a witness who was her professor at the University and how bright she was and all the many allegedly positive attributes that were hers; how she was respected in her community; what a religious person she is.

He continued to state how dangerous the prisoners could be; how firm one has to be with them; how "kind and caring" she was to enter prison nursing and how she allegedly financially supported a Biafran child by sending money overseas. When the good attorney was finished with his arguments Beatrice Blufton's image was indeed that of a very unusual human, of a true Angel of Mercy.

The prosecutor presented his case in a very logical fashion citing all of the circumstances in the prison which were not conducive to a safe environment for prisoners. He explained that surveillance and caution were indeed necessary and that "healthy" precautions should have been taken to insure that the safety of the prisoner in question would have been assured. He saw no reason whatsoever why Nurse Blufton neglected the prisoner/patient. He should have been tended to immediately and without hesitancy. He certainly was not dangerous, was semi-conscious, could not move his body, was totally helpless. His vital signs should have been immediately taken; the physician should have been called at once, and the ambulance should have been there instantly. There was no reason for the neglect of a man who could have been saved. What the guards did or did not do to this poor human being had nothing to do with the neglectful, cruel, unprofessional behavior of RN Blufton. He further pointed out that the guards were not here on trial – that this is the hearing for her, a graduate nurse. Only that aspect that belongs to her is coming under consideration not what the guards did or did not do. The prosecutor further stated that the nurse was not in any danger from a man who had labored breathing, a man who was barely alive, a helpless human being.

Rebuttels between Blufton's attorney and the prosecutor ensued; extraneous circumstances were brought in by the defense; a church witness for Blufton testified about her "moral character" and questions were posed by members of the Hearing Panel. Technical questions about physiology, timing, heart rates, etc. were posed. A query was made about the relationship that the Respondent Blufton had with the prisoners, with the guards and with this particular prisoner. The Nurse was asked about her education, her background, what her grades in professional school were. She was even questioned about her parents, her siblings and what her outlook about sustaining life are. What she verbalized and what her true feelings were and what she exhibited in this situation and the treatment of the late prisoner were divergent and were incongruent. There was much that remained questionable and unspoken.

The defense attorney summarized his arguments by stating that this hard working professional nurse had been placed in a very precarious position. He emphasized that she is a church going person of good moral character, that she worked with very hard core criminals, that she did not cause the death of this inmate; that the guards were responsible for the condition of this man; that they should have taken precautions not to have permitted the other prisoners to harm him, nor should they have been engaged in possibly further physically abusive behavior toward him which possibly caused the damage he sustained to his body. He went on to state that the Nurse had to be in good standing with the guards lest she be injured by prisoners. She needed protection from the guards or her existence could be jeopardized. He spoke about her "clean" record as a nurse and her generosity as exemplified by her financial support of a Biafran child. He concluded by requesting that no disciplinary action be taken against this woman.

The Prosecutor concluded with his argument. He reviewed her actions in the situation at hand: Nurse Blufton showed an extreme lack of caring and allowed a man to die, a man who could have been saved given the proper medical attention. He pointed out the severe neglect with which she practiced her profession; that she paid no attention to the patient, that she wasted a considerable time before she even made an effort to take his vital signs, that she had no concern about the pain and agony that he experienced, the fear that no doubt permeated his being as he was attempting to breathe. He urged the jury panel to exact the discipline that she deserved and that her actions required; that she should not be permitted to continue her practice as nurse under the circumstances as exhibited by her conduct which resulted in the wrongful death of a patient/ a human being!

This situation was taken very seriously by the "Jury" panel. After all witnesses had been called and concluding remarks were made by both the defense and the prosecution, the deliberations were held and were complicated ones. It was felt that this woman should definitely not ever return to a prison situation where she has no supervision. Although much discussion ensued both pro and con the revocation of her ability to practice nursing, the ultimate edict was to suspend her license for one year with the addendum that she will have to take a course in emergency care.

Eugenia L. is a tall imposing looking licensed practical nurse who has practiced her profession for fifteen years. She was generally cheerful, polite to the patients that were under her care, had behaved in a mature responsible manner and was well liked by her professional peers.

Within recent weeks prior to the incident that we will here describe, Nurse "Eugie," as her friends called her, seemed "not to be herself." She looked depressed and her pace was slower than it had been; she was a little late in meting out the prescriptions to her charges and what once had been a caring concerned person had changed. She furthermore was disinterested in her surroundings and had retreated into her inner being.

This attitude followed a number of months after she had lost her ten year old child. (The child had died in an accident at a time of day when her mother, Nurse Eugie was working in her capacity as nurse).

On April second, six months after her child's death Eugenia was found on the floor of the ladies room in an unconscious state with a syringe at her side. She had apparently administered a controlled substance to herself. She was bleeding from the right arm on the side where the syringe had fallen to the floor. A white substance was observed in the tubing of the syringe which was dripping unto the tiles of the bathroom. "Eugie" seemed disoriented and in no position to continue ministering to her patients. When she was aroused by one of her colleagues she could not remember where she was or what had occurred shortly before she fell. The staff that saw her in this state was afraid for her and felt that she was in a poor condition, unable to control her physical being, as well as her emotional state. In spite of having been "caught in the act" she staunchly denied that she was using drugs that were not prescribed for or given to her. They belonged to the hospital and specifically to a patient.

This nurse on various occasions while employed at the current hospital had stolen the controlled drug Demerol for her personal use. No physician had ever prescribed Demerol for Eugenia, thus she ingested this medication without a prescription for this item. She had diverted this drug from a patient for whom it had been prescribed by his medical doctor. In addition she falsified the particular patient's record for whom the medication had been intended. Additionally she continued to falsify the record by documenting that she had dispensed the afore mentioned medication after the patient was no longer in the hospital.

It was also discovered that the Nurse in question diverted controlled drugs from other patients and fraudulently documented that these medications were administered. When "Eugie's" fraudulent behavior was uncovered she denied that the occurrences had taken place. She even denied that some of the signatures were hers in the medical chart. It took much investigating and much confronting before this woman admitted that the initials on the charts were hers. Nurse Eugenia was charged with three specifications by a preponderance of the evidence and she was found guilty!

All three specifications of the charges had been proven without a doubt and beginning with the first specification as follows:

The five member nurse board panel concluded that the respondent Eugenia was clearly impaired while she was at work when she was rendered unconscious during her shift, by a self injected drug. After she was revived, she was unable to complete her nursing duties. She had to leave work and her responsibilities, because of the use of the drug.

The second specification was that Nurse Eugenia withdrew and diverted Demerol on six different dates, but did not administer any of this drug to the patients involved, nor 'wasted' any amount of the drug, i.e., it means she did not discard it because it was no longer needed or useful for the alleged patients. In effect this nurse stole the Demerol for her own use during a relatively short period of time.

The third specification of charges alleges that Eugenia willfully made a false report by documenting, on six different dates and occasions that she had withdrawn the Demerol for specific patients. As the respondent knew, she had not withdrawn the Demerol for any of the patients in question. In the case of patient X, the patient had already been discharged from the hospital before Eugenia had withdrawn the Demerol; In regard to patient Y, she was not even assigned to render nursing care to the patient, and in another patient case (Z) the patient's doctor had not prescribed

Demerol. During the time that the nurse withdrew Demerol for the patients in question, not any of them had received the drug. Eugenia therefore committed the alleged unprofessional conduct by creating the fraudulent record of "dispensing," which falsely showed that the Demerol was dispensed for use by these specific patients without actually receiving this medication.

After much discussion and contemplation of the professional misconduct of Eugenia, the five board members made the following determination: The respondent is guilty of professional misconduct on many specific instances (as documented). As previously shown, respondent abused her position as a licensed practical nurse in order to steal drugs for her own use.

It was therefore unanimously recommended that Eugenia's license as a licensed practical nurse in the State of practice be suspended, upon each of the first, second and third specifications of the charges of which respondent has been found guilty, as stated, suspensions to run concurrently, until such time as respondent successfully completes a course of treatment as follows:

Eugenia shall enroll in a drug abuse program, to be chosen by her after obtaining prior written approval from the State Education Department, for evaluation, and any necessary treatment, and/or referral, all at the respondent's expense, and shall cooperate fully with and participate in said Department approved drug abuse program.

Shall successfully complete said drug abuse program and be found by said program to be fit to practice the profession of nursing.

After receipt and proof from respondent of the purported successful completion of the aforesaid program and of the finding by the program that she is fit to practice the profession of nursing, all of such proof is to be forwarded to the Director, Office of Professional Discipline, State Education Dept. and if the Director is satisfied that respondent has successfully completed said program and found by said program to be fit to the practice the profession of nursing, the Director shall notify respondent of the termination of the suspension of her license and the effective date thereof.

Upon the termination of the suspension of the respondent's license, respondent be placed on probation for two years. The respondent shall be subject to random drug testing, be restricted from being able to obtain and administer controlled substances, and remain free from drug abuse.

Latoya, a slim attractive thirty eight year old registered nurse had worked for many years in the dialysis unit in a large urban hospital. She seemed to be proficient and knowledgeable in many aspects of hospital work. She especially liked the nephrology department with its adjacent dialysis division. The only problem that could be found regarding this RN is that she occasionally appeared a few minutes late at work. She was skilled in handling her patients needs and complaints and she was well liked by the majority of them.

Two years prior to this writing a severe situation occurred involving two patients on nurse Latoya's unit. She was on that day the charge nurse for her Department. Latoya was found to have been aware that no pulse could be detected for the two patients and she observed air in the patients dialysis tubing. Both patients experienced cardiac arrest and died that day. The situation developed because of the improper administration and monitoring of I.V. (intravenous) medication by another nurse. Latoya and another nurse were found to have been present during efforts to resuscitate the patients. After the patients became pulse-less, Latoya failed to inform any of the physicians on the cardiac resuscitation team promptly. Additionally she did not make anyone on the medical team aware that air had infiltrated the patients dialysis tubing. Both patients died of an air embolism.

Additionally it was noted that on another occasion when this RN was on duty a similar situation had occurred as the aforementioned, only in another hospital. While employed on a hospital hemo-dialysis unit, she was responsible for a dialysis patient. It was found that, at the conclusion of the patient's dialysis, the patient was unconscious, appeared very pale and had a weak pulse. It was found that the Nurse

Latoya, without first thoroughly assessing the patient or informing a physician of the patient's condition, she permitted said patient to be removed from a mechanical ventilator and transferred to another floor of the hospital. The patient died as a result of the removal of the ventilator, together with the transfer of the patient, with a considerable delay, from the one location, one floor to the other, without the mechanical device in place. Latoya was thus found negligent on more than one occasion and her license was revoked.

Thirty seven year old Licensed Practical Nurse James Conner came before the nurse board panel because he had been charged with practicing the profession of nursing with gross negligence by a preponderance of the evidence. He is a fairly attractive man with long light brown hair, an ill kempt mustache and goatee who appeared very casually dressed in a light colored sweat suit with a golf player insignia in both front and back. His tennis shoes made a squeaking sound as he entered the hearing room with a hesitant gait. Through previous experience we learned that he had been "invited" on two previous occasions to come before the Board to confront the issues in question. He did not choose to appear on those occasions to face his problems. This, the third time, he reluctantly accepted to appear. The members of the hearing panel as well as the administrating officer, the prosecutor and the court reporter had just about given up and were ready to proceed without him when Mr. Conner made his entrance.

James had been employed by Haven Hill Nursing Home for eight years on the three to eleven P.M. shift and had performed adequately until the charge of gross negligence had been leveled against him by the facility.

One of his patients, Helen Dietrich, an eighty seven year old very frail woman measured over 550 on her blood glucose level. Seeing this he did not chart this situation, did not notify his supervisor immediately, nor the physician and decided to take no action. An hour later he took matters into his own hands and administered an inappropriate dose of medication to Helen. Her body responded by an increased level of glucose in her system. He next proceeded to take seven more samples of blood within a very short period of time to determine whether the glucose level was responding to the non controlled substance that he had administered. Ultimately the RN supervisor learned of the situation and Mrs. Dietrich in a very poor physical condition, near death, was transferred to a local hospital. Fortunately for all concerned the patient lived but not without damaging effects.

Jim knew the appropriate procedures and contingencies but failed to follow them. Since he brought no attorney to assist him in explaining his actions he was his own defendant during the hearing. At the rate of upward of one hundred fifty dollars an hour for legal services he could not afford this "luxury." He alleged that he attempted to locate his supervisor but could not find her. Eventually, much later, when he did see her she directed him not to record anything regarding this situation in the medical chart. He further stated that he knew the condition of his patient and that she had probably over eaten on starches and fruits which caused the problem; perhaps someone had given her candy. He continued to say that he had experience with this frail elderly woman and that her glucose level would eventually "spiral downward." He insisted that the RN supervisor was not on the premises when he searched for her or that possibly she was sleeping somewhere in the building. He did not telephone the physician in charge since he did not want to step over his authority because he did not want to face "repercussions," regardless of the outcome for Mrs. Dietrich. He staunchly insisted that he had brought her glucose level down at other times and that he had been certain that his ministrations would be effective once again.

Acting as his own attorney Mr. Conner brought in a witness – another LPN who attempted to validate everything that the respondent (defendant) had stated. The witness was of questionable character and although she attempted to sound authentic her appearance and reactions did not speak to this. Many of her statements were irrelevant to the situation under discussion. She talked about her four children, the fact that she was studying to be a registered nurse, also as an attorney and preparing for a Ph.D., all at the same time while she is out of work. When she was questioned

75

more closely she told the panel that she is "on disability" and that she is taking a correspondence course but is postponing it. She also said that she knows the Nursing Supervisor of the Haven Nursing Home and that this woman is incompetent and a prevaricator. She went on to say that it is improper to notify the patient's physician even if the Supervisor is unreachable. She continued at length to speak about her own late grandmother and how well she treated this woman and that the respondent was also good to her. Much that she said was free association and inconsequential to the situation at hand. Upon questioning the witness the board members received irrelevant answers and the Witness seemed to have a flight of ideas since she free associated and could not easily be kept on the topic at hand.

The prosecutor also had a witness. This woman, Joanne, was the Supervising Nurse of the Haven. Joanne staunchly denied that she was absent from the institution during the time that the respondent was looking for her and that she never left the premises while on duty. She went on to say that as soon as she learned of the incident she had the patient transferred to the hospital. She stated that she had not forbidden any nurse to call a physician if need be, although the protocol was for the RN supervisor to be responsible for this task. She informed the panel that she is no longer in the employ of the Haven Nursing Home but that she continues in her position as supervisor in another institution. This supervisor staunchly denied that she ever told the defendant that he should not document in the medical record. That it is in the role and the duty of every nurse to chart. The panelists asked many questions of this witness and she answered them without hesitation.

After a great deal of discussion, by the witnesses, the respondent and the prosecutor stating their case the three member panel decided that by a preponderance of the evidence the LPN was guilty of gross negligence. He had not followed the protocol of which he was aware. His nursing supervisor was in the building even if she had fallen asleep, it was his responsibility to awaken her under the circumstances. If by chance she could not be found he could have notified the patient's physician or the physician on call of the patient's condition. He apparently did not follow any of these steps and therefore endangered the life of a human being. The panel recommended that his license be suspended for a period of six months. Additionally he was directed to take a course in medical ethics as it pertains to nursing practice.

Ebonisha Lobaru an attractive, well groomed Registered Nurse was brought before the Nurse Board since she neglected her patients on numerous occasions by leaving her responsibilities long before her shift ended; by not administering the medications as prescribed, by absenting herself on at least eleven occasions when she was expected at work. She did not inform any one of the reason for her planned absences, not her supervisor, nor any staff members. She had worked diligently in her position in the psychiatric unit at Benton hospital for five years when these occurrences began. She had offered no explanations for her actions and was belligerent when questioned. When she appeared before the Nurse Board she was accompanied by her husband who attempted to act as her unlicensed "attorney." She had not brought an authentic lawyer to advocate for her.

When her unprofessional conduct was mentioned she became extremely angry and suspicious. She shouted that she was being persecuted because of her race and that "whities have it in" for her. She continued to insist that she is innocent of all charges. She further was adamant that there was a supervisor who was attempting to poison her in order to make space for a nurse that she, the supervisor, wanted to hire in the respondent's place. She claimed that this supervisor placed Ebonisha's lunch bag on the radiator of her office in order to add a drug that would ruin the respondent. This RN continued to allege that the then President of the United States had chosen her as a special envoy to "right things that were wrong" and that he cared for her in a special way. She went on to state that she was close to him in a very important baseball game in the New "World" Stadium.

Several witnesses testified regarding Ebonesha's "strange" behavior, her withdrawal from them. She recently ate alone, locked up in her office, was seen washing her hands repeatedly and being generally "different" than she had been in the past. She was apparently paranoid and created much havoc. She went so far as to inform the patients of her suspicions. After the first day of hearings the RN was asked to return for a second day so that a decision could be reached. A date was set for the convenience of the respondent, her spouse and defender, as well as the panel members and the prosecutor.

When the day in question came and the Board Members, etc. had assembled for the continuation of the session, the Respondent, Ebonesha was nowhere in sight. Instead she had written a letter to the Education Department's Nurse Board with a copy of each to the panel members. It was not a plea asking for the permission for RN L. to retain her license but a number of accusations of fiendish crimes committed on "my person" as follows: "Rape and sodomy, physical assaults to my body, sadistic forms of persecution and terror, destruction of my personal property, sexual harassment. I have not violated any form of nursing practice; I was maliciously locked up in an elevator and no one cared about my safety. While I was locked in the elevator a white male shouted: Bitch get out! My supervisor had the FBI threaten me; physical and psychological damage was done to me. I herewith demand justice!"

It was apparent to all of the panel members including the administrative officer, the prosecutor and all responsible parties that Ebonesha Lobaru is suffering from a serious mental disorder – a psychosis and cannot at this time be held responsible for her actions. It was decided to recommend suspension of her license until she has been treated successfully for her condition.

Looking at nurse "Ebby's" background we found a woman who was hard working, ambitious, wanted very much to be a nurse and was a very serious student while earning both her RN and a bachelors degree. She had grown up in the South, her mother had died when the child was three years old and her father abandoned her shortly thereafter. Various relatives and friends raised her in however fashion they could. Although she had little stability or love she was determined to change all that. She was equally determined to help others as she had wished they had done for her. During her adolescent years she fell in love with an eighteen year old school dropout who impregnated her. Soon thereafter he abandoned her. She visited a clinic and had an abortion for fear she would be "thrown out" of the temporary foster home in which she was living at the time. She managed to graduate from high school with good grades. She won a scholarship to a local nursing school and upon completion found work in a large eastern city. It was not long before she began taking night school courses at a University which ultimately led to her baccalaureate degree. During her early nursing career she was nurse for a male patient whom she ultimately married. She was the main bread winner for this gentleman since he was frequently unemployed. After a few years in the nursing field Ebonisha found the job that appealed to her, working with psychiatric patients. She felt that she could help them, to make them well, get love and gratitude in return and learn more about herself and her problems. The stress at home and the responsibilities seemed overwhelming at times. She often found that she could not concentrate, was forgetful and believed that strange things were happening to her. She felt unloved and used and felt dominated and disliked by her coworkers and supervisors. She had longed for the love that she had missed during her childhood years and could not regain her losses. She felt alone and unwanted. In her mind she was being persecuted which ultimately led to her psychotic break.

When looking at the perpetrators described here we see nurses who are the antithesis of that which the public expects of the nurses who they trust and rely on. They are people who have seriously deviated from the norm. They are individuals who went into a profession into which they do not fit and into which they do not belong. Some have arrived at this status accidentally and have made errors out of carelessness or inability to follow the expectations essential for a nursing career; others have willfully committed crimes against the patients that are under their care because of a lack of conscience or a lack of caring; yet others have failed because of ignorance, lack of thorough learning or education; yet others are suffering from uncontrolled addictions or a combination of the above. Often we cannot determine exactly what caused a nurse to behave in an unacceptable fashion. There are those among the perpetrators who are needy individuals who have lived in an emotionally barren existence from childhood on and exhibit their deprivations when the opportunity presents itself. There are those who may yearn to be loved and may in a conscious or unconscious way repeat that which was perpetrated upon them in their growing up years of their lives.

The reader must always remember there are deviants in every walk of life and in every profession. The majority of nurses are upstanding professionals who are a credit and a trustworthy segment of our population. Nursing has been chosen here because it is a very important licensed occupation and deviance in all aspects of the health care field can cause serious harm to patients and their families.

Chapter IV

Moral Character? Alcoholics, Drug Users and Thieves

We must first look at the definition of the meaning of moral character. Morality is described in Webster's dictionary as a doctrine or system of moral conduct. A moral character then is an individual whose behavior is ethical, honest and decent as interpreted by our culture. When an individual deviates from this tenet to an unacceptable extent he/she is considered immoral.

Nurses, like all of humanity are not immune to the vagaries of life that plague a segment of the population. Not unlike pharmacists and physicians they have easy access to drugs. The stress of the nursing profession is at times great and invites its weaker members to want to seek relief through self medicating, thus using anesthetics to relieve themselves of the pressures facing them.

It is essential here to stress that the majority of nurses are law abiding, and caring people who entered their profession to help the sick, the wounded, the people who are physically incapacitated and in distress. They are often exposed to the most difficult situations and are involved with unthinkable suffering. They see children and adults hurt and dying; they must assist with workers who have lost a limb; assist in stopping bleeding from severe wounds and must keep their wits about them while they are performing their life saving tasks. They are often the first on the scene. They cannot shy away from that which most ordinary people would avoid. Thus nursing, in the true meaning of the word takes an emotionally strong, knowledgeable, rational person who is caring, sympathetic and able to work under often extremely difficult circumstances and situations. It must be remembered that when we speak about deviant nurses we are here only discussing those nurses and situations who were unable to follow the path of the majority, those who succumbed to weaknesses not the truly dedicated nurses just described. The deviant nurse is one who for some reason, possibly lack of motivation, childhood upbringing, life circumstances, learning difficulties, personality problems, poor role models, etc. has committed the acts and or behaviors that will be described.

Forty year old Concetta "Connie" an attractive but obese woman was working in a nursing home for many years. She was very proud of her LPN (licensed practical nurse) license which she had earned a year after graduating from high school. Her grades were good and her techniques for dressing wounds, making beds, feeding, giving injections were excellent. She was friendly to her patients and was congenial with fellow staff members for whom she did many favors. She rarely refused her nursing colleagues when they needed someone to take their place, or fill some of their other responsibilities. She had a strong need to be liked and appreciated. When asked about her motivation for entering the field of nursing she stated that she wanted to help people who were in need. She especially expressed her love for the geriatric patients and had a tendency to "mother" them. She would patronize and direct them.

Connie alternated between working on the second shift from three to eleven p.m. and on the night shift. She preferred the latter since she had two adolescent children at home who needed supervision.

Over a considerable period of time patients and their families complained of missing items of clothing, snack items, money and other possessions that were kept in patients rooms. The clothing items were explained by way of the laundry – miss marked items, possibly stashed in other patients rooms or "just lost." Missing money was rationalized that other residents might have come into a particular room and helped themselves to the dollars. One day a very expensive diamond and emerald ring was missing from a woman's finger. The family of the patient was irate. They had seen it on their mothers hand the day before and when they returned it had disappeared. It was a night when Connie had been the nurse for the floor that the ring-less patient occupied. The aide, the cleaning help the nurse and others were questioned by the administration and no one seemed to know anything about the missing jewelry. The patient privately and fearfully told the director of nursing who interrogated everyone, that she had half awakened and was in a hypnogogic state when she felt someone twisting her heirloom off her finger. The thief had a difficult time removing it and it pained with every turn. The patient recalled saying "ouch" and saw the form of what she believed was the large body of nurse Connie. (Incidentally the patient pleaded that her name should not be mentioned in that connection because she was afraid of being abused if she was the complainant or the reporter). It was noticed that the patient had a red and swollen ring finger on her left hand. Nothing further was said to Connie but she was closely observed. For a time there was no theft. About a month after the ring theft other items of jewelry and new underwear were missing. Connie was surprised by the night aide as she removed a gold cross chain from the neck of a sleeping patient. The aide reported this incident and subsequently the nurse was removed from her job and ultimately brought before the Board of Nursing.

In looking at the background of Concetta we learned that she was an out of wedlock child of a woman who neglected Connie from the time she was very young. Her mother would go out with various boyfriends and locked the child into the apartment until she returned from her various dates. She would on occasion bring a male into the house and would openly engage in various sexual activities without regard for the little girl. When Connie was three one little brother was born and at age four and five she attained two more brothers. She recalled having to "baby sit" the younger ones and when she was six her mother produced yet another boy. Connie Kapsy frequently had to miss school because she had to take care of "the boys." The welfare department workers visited fairly frequently because the neighbors reported that children were left alone and the apartment where they lived was kept in disarray and "filth." Cockroaches were reported crawling out of the Kapsy apartment and at that point the children were removed. Connie remembers a little tiny brother who fell out of his high chair. Connie was alone and she attempted to pick up the crying baby but she did not have the strength to do so. She felt frightened and guilty when the welfare worker took him and later all of them away. She never knew what happened to the youngest baby but eventually surmised that he had been adopted. She grieved him for a long time and felt that she had caused the problems since she could not help him. There was never enough food in the Kapsy household and Connie often went hungry. She dreamed of food and being rich and getting all the ice cream that she could eat. She loved school and always felt bad when she could not attend due to having to play Mom for the remaining siblings. At age seven Connie was placed in a foster home. It was a poor solution to her problems. They did not feed her well and she sometimes had the chance to steal some food and gorge it down before the family caught and scolded her. Because of this she ultimately was removed and placed into a number of foster homes, none of which were acceptable as far as the child was concerned. Eventually as a later adolescent Connie returned home. By that time Ms. Kapsy was allegedly married to a man whom Connie called "Dad" and Ms. Kapsy had given birth to two daughters. There was now enough food in the house and Connie took advantage of it. She never seemed to get enough. She satisfied her emptiness with food and gained much weight in the process.

Connie was a good student in high school and at nineteen she received her Practical Nurse License. She had fulfilled her dream of finally being someone! She was able to mother people the way she had never been mothered; people would ask her for advice and she felt fulfilled. She worked hard and during her care giving experiences she met a young man who was unemployed to whom she was attracted. The two got married and had a son and daughter. Connie's husband never held a steady job and was without work most of the time and enjoyed drinking with his friends.

One day while at work Connie was called by the police to inform her that her mother and stepfather had been killed in an automobile accident. Connie was devastated. Aside from losing her only parent she was now responsible for raising her two teenage sisters.

Connie became angry and bitter but did not show this directly to her patients. She always smiled at them and seemed to be an exemplary care giver. Her inner life took a different turn. She was like two separate beings. She felt deprived and fated to take over great burdens. She resented anyone who had money, stability and earthly goods. When she stole she was convinced that she was entitled to have whatever she could have regardless of how the acquisitions were obtained. She believed that no one really understood her and she had to be her own "mother" – the mother that she had never had or experienced.

She became the pseudo mother of the old agers whom she served and the praise that she received from them felt good. At the same time she yearned for more concrete shows of affection from her charges. When they could not or would not give her material things to which she felt entitled, she helped herself without any moral flickers of conscience.

When Connie was ultimately confronted and terminated by her employer she was angry and outraged. When questioned she changed her story a number of times. At first she alleged that she meant to place the items in the institutions safe deposit box. Another time she insisted that she had merely taken the jewelry home to keep it safe for the patient and that she had intended to eventually return it. The only regret that she had regarding the theft was that she was "caught" and that her income had ceased and her nursing license was revoked.

Madeline Sommers, a licensed practical nurse, was convicted of committing acts constituting a crime under her State's law "within the purview and meaning of the State's Education Law." The conviction was for Petit Larceny.

The facts were that while working, for the "G" family the respondent did take, on several occasions, with the intent to permanently remove, from said residence certain sums of cash in excess of one thousand dollars, to which respondent knew she had no right to take and/or to permanently remove.

On May 7, 1997 respondent was, while on duty in the "G's" residence , surreptitiously seen by "G" family members (who had become concerned over the apparent disappearances of cash from the residence and who were observing through windows from the outside of said residence) taking sums of money which had been specifically secreted inside the premises. Said cash had been marked by the "G" family members.

As a result of said observations, the Town Police were called and respondent was arrested as she was leaving the "G" family residence.

Pursuant to a police search of respondent's handbag, conducted as a result of said arrest, respondent was found to have in her possession two hundred and fifty one dollars which were identified by "G" family members as being among the cash which had been secreted in the residence earlier in the day.

Ms. Sommers first job was working in a private household as an aide a few nights a week to assist the family in helping their elderly, eighty nine year old, frail mother. She continued this job on a more full time basis when she received her LPN license. This young woman was well liked by the patient as well as by Jane and Peter, her adult children. Madeline would always be on time, reliable and meticulous in her care giving responsibilities and was friendly and personable. In short, she seemed an ideal, sincerely caring individual. She was never hesitant to do "a little extra work" like doing laundry that Jane left for her, washing the bathroom and kitchen floors and keeping her patient clean, well fed and presentable.

On a number of occasions Jane noticed that there was money missing from the patient's home. It was money that was kept in a special place and used as needed. Sometimes it would accumulate to quite a sum especially when the social security check was cashed. The patient's life time habit was to keep a considerable sum of money in her home and she felt secure knowing that she would "never be in need and pay her just and honest debts" at any time without hesitation.

Madeline found the "stash" of large and small bills not long after she began working for the "G" family. Although Mrs. G, the patient was a very trusting woman her family was not. Mrs. G's eyesight was not too good, and she did not always know how much she owned and in what denominations. Madeline rationalized that she needed the money much more than her patient did. She also believed she was not earning as much as she should have and that therefore she deserved more. She felt no compunction about removing a large or some smaller bills at various times and was certain that no one would ever notice. She took the money always when Mrs. G and she were alone and most frequently when her patient was in bed and asleep. She felt in no danger of being observed and happy that she could buy what she wanted and desired for an amount that she had not specifically worked for. She also experienced a certain exhilaration when she felt the "bills" in her hand. As time went on she felt more and more secure in her successful performance of dispossessing the woman of the funds that were "gathering dust" and that she was convinced that the patient did not need.

Ultimately when the respondent was arrested and found guilty she had to make full restitution of the stolen funds. She was able to accomplish this within nine months of the aforementioned crime. She succeeded with very hard work, taking two menial jobs, sixteen hours per day, six days a week.

In addition to the criminal charges she also lost her nursing license which was revoked.

Four years later Ms. Sommers appeared before the nurse board having gone back to school and passed all courses and the examination for the RN degree. She was eager to return to her profession. She seemed truly remorseful for what she had done and related her past conviction openly and sincerely.

Based upon Ms. Sommer's testimony and stipulation to the facts contained in the specification of professional misconduct, and respondent's admission of guilt to said specification there was no remaining question to respondent's culpability in this matter.

Arguments pro and con allowing this person to have her license and to practice as a registered nurse were made. One statement was that the purpose of punishment is not to just punish and deter the wrongdoer but to also deter other health care professionals who might be tempted to steal from patients or clients. It is to send a stern message to keep others from engaging in misconduct.

Another argument in behalf of the respondent was that she should get her license and be permitted to practice since she admitted her guilt, explained her sorrow and remorse for having violated a sacred trust. She had already paid her debt to society and to the "G" family specifically.

While the members of the Nurse Board Panel found merit in both arguments that a penalty should be given which is both appropriate for the offense committed and in addition is responsive to the needs of the profession and the consuming public. Into consideration taken was the fact that the respondent's misconduct occurred over four years ago. Full restitution was made to the victims and no further misconduct, related or unrelated to the proven misconduct has been proven or alleged. In the interim period Ms. Sommers has successfully completed all necessary course work and examination for the registered nurse exam. Co-workers in her jobs, neighbors and others including some nurses submitted supportive affidavits or personally came forward to testify on respondent's behalf. A therapist, licensed social worker, testified based on his contacts with Madeline that it was not likely that she would repeat her prior misconduct. While there is no question that the respondent's misconduct was and is a very serious matter deserving of an appropriate sanction, especially considering the professionally intimate nature of the nurse- patient relationship it was the opinion of the panel that the respondent is not likely to again repeat said misconduct. There were also no records of prior deviant acts by this woman.

Although a determination of guilt was apparent recommendations and an appropriate penalty were made:

- No duties in private households were to be taken for the foreseeable future.
- After a period of six months respondent would be able to practice as an RN
- Respondent was to perform one hundred and fifty hours of community service.

Liller Kinton came before the three member nurse board since she wanted to be permitted to practice as a Licensed Practical Nurse. In order to qualify for licensure she was aware that she had to fulfill various requirements, one of which is that the applicant must be of good moral character. This is at times difficult to ascertain and it is the responsibility of the applicant to bring testimony, references, possible witnesses and sources to attest to that matter. The burden of proof is on the individual desiring to be in the profession to which they have aspired.

Ms. Kinton was not represented by an attorney. The facts that were presented to the Board were as follows: Six years previous to this date Liller was convicted of embezzlement by the United States District Court. She was subsequently sentenced to remain in the custody of the U.S. Marshal on the day of sentencing and thereafter to a five year term of supervised release and was required to make restitution in the amount of $20,400 at the rate of two hundred dollars per month until the debt was cleared.

She had plead guilty to the charge and admitted that she had over a period of fourteen months while employed by a large bank, taken money for her own use which belonged to a customer.

When she testified before the Nurse Board she related that she was eighteen years old at the time that she worked at the Bank and that this employment was her first full time job since graduating from high school. She enjoyed the position of teller and was happy. Previous to that she had held a number of part time jobs to buy those items which she felt she needed. She stated that she was not certain why she stole from the Bank except that she saw all this money coming in and she felt poor in relationship to what she saw coming in and out of the many accounts. She had no valid excuse for her actions and was aware that at eighteen years of age she was considered to be an adult and responsible for her own behavior. She did admit that her best friend at that time pressured her to violate a customer's account and convinced her that she would not be discovered and that there would be no consequences for her actions.

After working at the Bank she left her employment and began college. A few months after that Liller received a telephone call from her old place of employment regarding a discrepancy in a customer's account. Before the commencement of the criminal matter Liller admitted to having committed the theft and agreed to make restitution in the increments as demanded. The realization had come to her that she could not "cover up" what she had done and that it was she who had committed the crime as stated.

Within the subsequent year she applied and was accepted into an LPN School where she completed the program. She worked very hard during the course of her one year program and graduated with honors. She especially had enjoyed the clinical aspect of her training, liked the hospital and nursing home part and confirmed her desire to be a nurse. She enjoyed the care giving, providing patient care and feeling good about helping human beings. It was a very positive experience for her.

Ms. Kinton stated that she now questions her own motivation and mind set that motivated her to commit the crime which resulted in her conviction. She recognizes now that she caused pain to the woman from whose account she embezzled the money and is remorseful for it. In spite of the fact that she has made restitution and is still in the process of fulfilling the remainder of her obligation she understands that it cannot pay for the pain that she caused her victim.

Liller testified that she has learned and has become a more mature and responsible person since her employment at the Bank. She further realized that it is wrong to do illegal acts and to disregard the consequences of such acts.

She informed the Board members that she has since had a son which has aided in her maturity and made her a more responsible human being. She cannot imagine repeating her former conduct, nor of jeopardizing her baby as the result of deviant behavior.

Liller believes she is a good person and has always been a good person but a foolish one who has made a mistake that she wishes she could change. She explained that she never considered herself evil and not one to steal.She was tempted by the proximity of cash at the Bank of large sums of money. She admitted that she was immature, irresponsible and did not consider the impact of her actions on her victim. She denied that she would ever again steal, even if she knew she would not be caught and cited an example that she returned money dropped by a co-worker. She could have pocketed the money and not be detected.

Liller stated if she were permitted to proceed to be licensed, she would take a nursing refresher course to update her skills and she would work as a certified nursing assistant for a three month period to retain and relearn whatever techniques were needed to be a good and skilled nurse.

The following determinations were made and conclusions drawn:

- The applicant has been forthright in accepting responsibility for her wrongdoing and by admitting her guilt and agreeing to repay the monies she embezzled. She appears sincere in her expression of remorse for the pain that she inflicted on the victim of the crime.

- The applicant, having graduated from nursing school with honors , plans to pursue a degree program to obtain training as a registered professional nurse, demonstrating a committed, goal oriented effort to put her past behind her and continue with a productive and worthwhile life.

In Liller's favor are her very supportive family. Her mother is always ready to take over the majority of the care of the applicant's child. In addition to child- care the woman's mother has provided significant encouragement to study nursing and has helped her financially as well.

The three members of the "jury" felt that the wrongdoing was a single, aberrant event perpetrated by a young woman who was too immature and irresponsible to consider the consequences, both for the victim of her crime and for herself. It should be noted that the federal court struggled with federal sentencing guidelines to insure that Liller would not be incarcerated.

Since committing the crime and during the intervening years, Ms. Kinton paid for her malfeasance, gained a nursing education with honors, gave birth to a son and developed an enhanced sense of right and wrong and compassion for others.

After examining the factors set out in Corrections Law it was concluded that licensure of Ms. Kinton as a licensed practical nurse would not involve an unreasonable risk of harm to the public. After extensive examination of all matters involved and consideration it was unanimously agreed by the three Board members that the applicant had sufficiently fulfilled the moral character requirement. It was agreed that the applicant's application to be a licensed practical nurse be granted.

Rowena Andress was called before the Nurse Board's "jury" panel because she had falsified her application for becoming a licensed practical nurse. 1. The question in the application was the following: "Have you ever been convicted of a crime (felony or misdemeanor) in any state or country?" Rowena responded with a "no." 2. In addition she failed to disclose that she had been convicted in a County Court of Law of Criminal Trespass in the Second Degree, a class A misdemeanor in violation of the State's penal law. 3. On the same date she failed to disclose that she also pleaded guilty to Petit Larceny, a class A misdemeanor. She was found guilty of all charges and had received three years of probation at that time. All of these charges had occurred four years prior to her application for her LPN license.

An investigator from the State of practice telephoned the Respondent, Rowena and invited her to attend the session before the Board. She was also sent a letter notifying her of the date of the conference. She did not verbally refuse to appear and consented to be heard. When the date of the hearing in September of 2000 arrived and the members of the State Board were assembled Ms. Andress did not appear. No excuse was sent although she had five weeks to prepare for this meeting. She was telephoned repeatedly, offered no excuse and several times did not answer her telephone. Ultimately she accepted a date and again did not appear. Two years later and with the agreement of the LPN she made a date and was a "no show." This time the members of the Nurse Board Panel together with the prosecuting attorney, the administrating officer for the State and the Investigator proceeded without Rowena. The Investigator who had telephonically interviewed the client informed the participants of the meeting of the occurrences that had taken place to create the problem before them.

Rowena had deliberately falsified her records and had subsequently under false premises obtained her nursing license. The other charges dealt with her breaking and entering a home and stealing various objects which she wanted and which allegedly had at one time been hers. Her current significant other had donned gloves to steal these objects and with the help of the Respondent had left that house in "shambles" searching for the objects of her choice. She had been discovered by neighbors of the home, the police were called and she, as well as her significant other, were apprehended and subsequently taken before the court.

Much discussion ensued among the members of the panel. It is true that she had been practicing nursing for a number of years. Since that practice was built on dishonesty all involved feared for the welfare of the vulnerable clients whom she was serving. Theft was rampant in the nursing home where Rowena was employed. The question had whether she had been involved in the disappearance of goods belonging to the residents of that institution. When her past record was discovered she seemed to have no remorse. She also had every opportunity to appear and to explain herself and defend the accusations and determinations made in the three "crimes" of which she was found guilty. Instead of that she decided to play the proverbial ostrich and ignore the requests of the Nurse Board. She had the opportunity to prove that since the time that she was convicted a number of years had passed and she had redeemed herself and had matured into an honest reliable human being. She could have brought references, character witnesses and remorse for her past history. None of this happened.

After much discussion and hours of "pro and cons" the members of the nurse board decided to suspend Ms. Andress' license for a period of one year, have her successfully pass an ethics course and charge her a fine of $500. This determination was a unanimous one by all three panel member participants.

Janzetta Jones a registered nurse had been practicing in Creation Hospital for five years with a leave of six months in between to deliver the last of her four children. She had been in several other hospitals earlier in her career and had left positions very speedily at times. References in the past places were meaningless and one of the hospitals in which she was employed gave a strange response concerning the reason for her quick departure. She had some excellent references from friends but nothing substantial from former employers.

It appeared that in one of the places, a nursing facility where Respondent worked very briefly, had a major theft reported in which a considerable sum of money and an expensive diamond heirloom ring had disappeared from one of the patient's who had been Janzetta's responsibility.

She had been found guilty and terminated from Creation Hospital four years ago at the time of this writing and came before the three member panel to attempt to get her license back. The reasons for her dismissal was that she ignored a patient whose oxygen equipment was not in place – she had been without the nasal tube for an extended period of time; she also, during that same early morning shift had failed to properly monitor her patient while administering the medication Vancomycin through an I.V. (intravenous device). Thus the medication drained completely out of the bag and air infiltrated the patient's I.V. tubing. Ms. Jones did not call the physician and her patient subsequently died of an air embolism.

On another day she had moved a seriously ill Aids patient out of his room for a risky procedure and without checking his pulse rate, respiration or his blood pressure. She disconnected his respirator before the transport. There was some delay in getting the patient to his destination and subsequently during the ride to another floor for the procedure, the patient died..

There were many specifications of negligence and incompetence in the case of Ms Jones and her professional responsibilities. She had failed to satisfy her responsibilities, had not communicated with the doctors who therefore could not determine the correct course of treatment. Appropriate care to the patient had obviously not been given. It had been the determination of the Board of Nursing that Janzetta's practice as a registered professional nurse posed a danger to the public. She had demonstrated an inability to make sound decisions under pressure and presented herself as a nurse who is unsure of herself, incompetent, acted in a rash manner without regard for the safety of her patients. She also refused to accept responsibility for her actions and continued to attempt to blame others for her deeds or lack thereof.

It was unanimously recommended that the respondent's license to practice as a registered professional nurse be revoked. If she ever was to have her license reactivated she would have to take a refresher course in a number of areas including dialysis, hemodialysis and the tubing that is a part of the administering of the patient care, all of the equipment, how it is used and what to do in case of failure. She needed a course in emergency care; needed to deal with intubation, use and hazard of ventilator operations, oxygen equipment; tracheotomy care; ethics, etc.

It was four years later that Ms. Janzetta Jones appeared before the panel of Board members for a moral character hearing in an attempt to have her license reinstated.

She came with her attorney, brought proof of the many courses she had taken together with many letters of reference. She also brought verification of the grades she had obtained. She had passed with high grades and recommendations.

The attorney brought to light that at the times that she had been accused of the errors that she made she was alone and the floor on which she worked was not covered adequately with professional personnel. She denied any criminal history and this was confirmed by her lawyer.

In addition to the many courses and workshops that she had taken was one in pharmacology, one in geriatric care, another in medical equipment and their usages. There were several courses in emergency room care and dialysis administration. Her letters of reference included those from professionals she had worked with and for: Physicians, nursing supervisors, colleagues and friends. They included such statements as: Janzetta was very dedicated and diligent; that she would not purposely commit any act of negligence or incompetence. This was written by a physician who strongly recommended that Ms. Jones license be restored. Another reference stated that she knew the Nurse for fifteen years. She had professional experience with her when they both worked in one of the hospitals. She alleged that Janzetta was diligent, caring and dependable. This nurse had some knowledge about the issues that generated Ms. Jones revocation. She swore under oath that having worked with J.J. she had never had a problem with her and that she followed orders without argument. She felt that the subject worked with competence. Another reference letter stated that the respondent was reliable and rarely late or absent from work. Yet another letter stated that she knew Janzetta to be a good supervisor with strong clinical skills. The reference further stated that she did not know the reason for the respondent's revocation. Another physician, a cardiologist, wrote a reference stating that he has known the subject for fifteen years. He felt she was an excellent nurse. He was unaware of the specifics why the subject lost her license. This physician stated that he saw Ms. Jones approximately one year ago when she asked for an affidavit of support. He could not recall when he last saw her before then. He believed that this woman is of good moral character. At the same time he stated that if there were any doubt she should be closely observed for a period of one year to ascertain that she is performing with competence and compassion.

Janzetta was questioned by the panel how she financially supported herself during the period of revocation. In the beginning she took on some menial jobs on a temporary basis. Later she decided to concentrate on her courses and for a considerable length of time she replied that she has not worked. She receives an income from Social Security Disability. She has had a kidney transplant together with diabetes and was in the process of recovering.

After much thought given to this situation and much discussion the panel members agreed that Ms Janzetta Jones had carried out all recommendations. She has exhibited sincere remorse for the occurrences which resulted in her dismissal and subsequent penalty. She together with her attorney felt that much of what had happened was to a large extent the fact that she was alone without adequate help.

All three members of the Board panel decided to recommend that the Respondent's license to practice the profession of nursing be restored.

Ron and Jane Lucretia both Registered Nurses, a husband and wife "team" were employed in a large urban hospital in a medium sized city. Ron was taking care of Lester M. a very ill oxygen dependent tube fed total care patient. He had the night shift while his wife worked the day shift. The couple were especially interested in this man since his family was wealthy and they believed that they could earn some additional money from taking special care of him. They eventually approached the wife as well as the son and daughter of this man with the suggestion that they would give him better care if they took care of him in the gentleman's own home. They stated that costs would be reduced; that he would not have to end up in a nursing facility and that he would no doubt improve, getting the total attention of the Lucretia's. They sounded so enthusiastic and damned institutional care so much that the M's were eventually convinced that they followed the advice of the two nurses. The patient was subsequently moved out of the hospital with all of the necessary equipment to enable him to remain among the living. The couple took turns giving attention to Mr. M who slept much of the time. The couple had quit their job at the hospital and took twelve hour shifts thus covering the twenty four hour period. It did not take long before they were both collecting a very excellent salary. In addition they helped themselves to cash that Mrs. M. kept in a home safe. The couple somehow learned the combination of the safe and realized that there were large bills to be had, especially when large pension and other checks arrived, cashed and the moneys were stashed away "securely." Frequently when RN Jane had the night shift she would fall asleep. During one such night the oxygen equipment was not functioning and it was not noticed by the sleeping nurse. By morning Lester had expired from oxygen deprivation. The wife had come into the bedroom at seven a.m. and found her husband dead. Jane attempted to cover up the situation but did not succeed. The son had earlier believed that he discovered that money had been missing from the safe and was beginning to mistrust the two care givers. He had for a few weeks counted the funds in the safe and noticed that large sums were unaccounted for. When questioned the couple denied any wrong doing. Having marked a number of the larger bills, several were found in Ron's wallet.

When the patient's wife telephoned him with the sad news of the death he came immediately and noticed that no air was coming from the oxygen equipment. He questioned the nurse who had obviously paid little attention to her patient and failed to see him struggling for air.

When Jane was questioned she contradicted herself many times. Her husband attempted to say that the patient's wife was suffering from "senility" (Mrs. M. was in reality a very lucid woman) and that she was herself responsible from the missing money and that she perhaps had something to do with the flawed oxygen situation as well.

Upon the advice of the family physician as well as their attorney both the Health Department and the State Board of Nursing were notified of the situation.

A hearing was scheduled and held. Witnesses were called to testify for and against the two RN's and by a preponderance of the evidence it was found that the couple were guilty as charged. They had not only neglected the patient but had been engaged in theft. It was recommended unanimously that the license for both individuals be revoked. In addition they were charged a fine of five thousand dollars and a repayment to the family of another five thousand. At the time of this writing it is uncertain whether these perpetrators will come before a criminal court. (The patient's wife requested that this not take place.)

Letisha Green worked at the Avenue Nursing Facility, a two hundred bed long term care institution for chiefly elderly clients. She had been a Licensed Practical

Nurse for a period of three years and seemed to be reliable and responsible for the first two years of her employment. She worked the night shift and liked this since she was independent of "excessive" supervision. Within the past year she had appeared more tired and not as cheerful as usual. She was more impatient with the residents and hurried through the tasks that were assigned. Ms. Green felt over burdened since she had three adolescent children at home and no one to assist her since she was a single mother without much support.

One day while at work she "passed out" in one of the patient's rooms and was discovered by one of the aides. It took some time before she could be aroused. The night supervisor was called and it appeared that she was suffering from drug intoxication. A report was made and the nurse was sent home. Since there was no absolute diagnosis and no physician was called she returned to work for her next shift two days later. For a time there did not seem to be a severe problem. It was discovered that Nurse Letisha was confiscating medication from the patients and diverting them for her own use. A shortage of drugs were noticed and there was little explanation for this. It always occurred when Ms. Green was on duty. She was carefully observed by the night supervisor after a number of suspicious episodes. She had access to the narcotics closet and had the keys. When she was found taking narcotics by her supervisor and confronted she admitted that she had been diverting the drugs for some time. Tearfully she described her struggles and confessed that she was addicted and felt unable to control the habit. She did not seem to have any feeling for the patients who were suffering from serious often terminal illnesses and who were in excruciating pain and needed the drugs that she stole.

Letisha was terminated from her place of employment and subsequently reported to the State Education Department's Nurse Board. She was given the choice of giving up her license temporarily until she had completed a licensed Drug and Alcoholism Rehabilitation Program or whether she wanted to undergo a disciplinary session. She chose the Rehabilitation Program. This gave her the opportunity to have her license returned as soon as she and the program felt secure that she would remain drug and/or alcohol free.

   Dedrianna Latt, a sixty year old licensed practical nurse had worked at a large psychiatric center where she was responsible for a number of children and adolescents. She had long been suspected of being a bit "loopy" by her fellow workers. It was suspected that she was either a "silent alcoholic" or taking drugs that were readily available to her. Although she was seen "discarding" left over prescription drugs from the narcotics cabinet no one ever saw her placing them into her mouth. One of the other female attendants believed that she gave herself an injection but this was not reported until after she had been involved in the incidents which brought her before the State Education's hearing panel. The reasons for the disciplinary meetings were as follows: Ms Latt had pushed a twelve and a half year old male psychiatric patient repeatedly. The child, Manuel was upset with a young female patient who had thrown clothing and bedding around Manuel's room. Manuel ran up to the young girl Jill in the hall outside of his room, punched and hit her, throwing her to the floor and kicking her. The LPN seeing this called out to Manuel to stop assaulting Jill. She demanded that he go into his room and to close the door behind him. Manuel did not respond to this command and Ms. Latt separated the two children, and holding the boy around his shoulders led him to his room forcibly. Manuel continued to rage verbally and flailing he stated: "I fuckin gonna kill her. I'm gonna punch her teeth down her throat," etc. The screaming did not seem to end. He continued statements regarding bodily harm, did not respond to Nurse Latt's requests to straighten up his room. She allegedly tried repeatedly to redirect the boy but to no avail. In the interim other nurses assisted Jill and got her out of the vicinity where Manuel was shouting expletives and threats. He next shoved past Dedrianna and attempted to get out of the room. He issued threats for Jill and to the Nurse. Pushing him back onto the bed did not help since he got up again and again and he was extremely difficult to detain. He screamed and pushed the Respondent unto the bed and in a loud raucous voice said: "Bitch if you don't get out of my way, I'm gonna fuck you up." He then swung at the woman, hitting her on the upper arm and attempted to push this large woman again and again. At that point the nurse pushed Manuel again and again, past his desk, into the bathroom door. Ms. Latt stepped into the hallway and was observed by another staff member. Curses and threats emanated from the mouth of the boy including a statement that he would report her to his supervisor for pushing and hurting him so hard. He in fact saw the nurse coordinator in the hall and screamed that Nurse Latt had hit him about the head and ear. This boy was clever enough to know that it was the policy of the institution not to allow punching or pushing of patients.

A memo was written by the nurse coordinator to the Director of Nursing about what she had heard and in part witnessed. She did state that she did not see the beginning of the altercation nor did she see which part of the body of Manuel had been punched by Nurse Latt.

When this case came before the "jury" panel of the Nurse Board it was agreed that Nurse Latt was guilty of punching the boy Manuel. Since it is the policy of the Psychiatric Hospital not to injure, punch, push or hit children nurse Latt had ignored that policy. She had physically engaged in such behavior. (She had known and been taught to better handle maladaptive behavior in children). At the time of the incident she had also been suspected of having had some "medication" which changed her mood that day and she was being closely observed by her supervisor for her mood changes and possible drug diversion.

Considering the circumstances in relationship to this situation the Nurse Board panel members unanimously imposed the following recommendations upon the Respondent:

The respondent's license to practice as a licensed practical nurse be suspended for three months for the charges for which this nurse has been found guilty. It was further agreed that the Nurse be fined five hundred dollars which must be paid before the suspension expires and prior to the time that the respondent can resume her profession as licensed professional nurse.

Dora Rapnow, registered nurse held the position of nursing supervisor in a large three hundred bed geriatric facility. She worked the night shift and frequently went from floor to floor making her presence known, speaking to the nurses and aides at their stations and seeing that "all is well and orderly." She went through this routine every night, appearing at specific times in each section like an automaton. She always seemed cheerful during the early part of the night. She was never seen between two and four A.M. but this was ignored by her supervisors until Nurse Rapnow was needed to arrange for a hospital transfer for two very acutely ill residents. An aide was sent from floor to floor, from section to section but Dora could not be found. The loudspeaker was finally utilized to alert the Nurse of the circumstances which needed her immediate assistance. (The supervisors were those designated in the policy and procedure code book to do the task of transfer). Even the noise of the loudspeaker had no effect. After an extensive search with no response, an LPN took matters in her own hands and telephoned the hospital and an ambulance to effect the transfer. Many minutes had passed and the two affected residents were in life threatening danger. One died an hour after entering the hospital.

The Nurse Supervisor appeared at four A.M. with glazed eyes and somewhat groggy. She insisted she was in the building and could not hear the microphone although she was not known to have a hearing problem.

It was after the afore- mentioned episode that unbeknown to Dora she was closely observed. She was seen opening the narcotics cabinet, popping something in her mouth, walking out to her car and curling up in the back seat. Exactly two hours later she returned and resumed her duties as before.

It was not long before she was called into a meeting with the Director of Nursing and the Administrator and terminated. They contacted the State Education Department's Nurse Board and a hearing was scheduled. Dora was given the opportunity to enter a Drug and Alcohol Recovery Program and to willingly enter rehabilitation, but she adamantly refused. When she was apprized of a hearing date before the panel she accepted, but a day prior to the session she alleged that she was too ill with a virus to attend. Two more times dates were made for t he respondents' appearance. Finally after the third offer she appeared. After a number of sessions before the jury panel with many witnesses for and against Ms. R's competency it was discovered that Ms. Rapnow was addicted to drugs and had been for some time. The episode which brought her to the attention of the Nurse Board was a blatant one. She had been very skilled in concealing her affliction. When she curled up in her car to sleep at the same time each night she had always followed the same routine: A pill from the narcotic closet, a little time elapse, a trip to her car where a small alarm clock was set to wake her from her slumber and back to work.

Despite the fact that her attorney pleaded her case, praising her many years as a "good and competent nurse," with many character references and nurse friends lauding her abilities and knowledge, the prosecutor had a strong case against her. He insisted that she could not function competently being a drug addict; that she was guilty of neglecting and being the major cause of the one patient's death and the worsening of the other resident's physical deterioration and subsequent mental suffering; that she did not carry out her duties as prescribed.

The Nurse was found guilty of negligence and petit larceny (theft of the drugs that she diverted for her own use) by preponderance of the evidence presented.

After much thought, discussion and contemplation the members of the Nurse Board panel recommended the following: A minimum of one year suspension of the respondent's license; an inpatient course of treatment in a qualified drug rehabilitation program; and a course of medical ethics. She would have to prove that she had successfully completed all requirements thus made and exhibit drug free behavior for a minimum of one year. Following her ultimate return of her license she would not be able to work nights and would need to have a work site supervisor to assist her in remaining drug free.

We have here shown a small number of nurses who are involved in theft, drug use and immoral conduct. Such behavior can be found in other professions, occupations and all walks of life. The public expects more from nurses and medical personnel than they do from the ordinary, sometimes unenlightened citizen. We judge nurses to be above the lay person, to have more knowledge related to health, to well being as well as to have more education. We hold nurses in high esteem, they are in a position to hold the key of life for the very vulnerable patients under their care. Most nurses are honorable people who ostensibly entered the profession of nursing because they are caring individuals who want to be of help, to assist in alleviating suffering and pain to make life better for those under their care.

One of the reasons for the relatively pronounced degree of drug use and theft perpetrated by the nurses described is that they have greater access to drugs and opportunity to obtain material goods than the average employee. It is also easier to find the deviant nurse since she is more vulnerable to scrutiny by supervisors and fellow employees. The ideal nurse then is one who is competent, cares for human beings, is knowledgable and scrupulously honest.

They must not use their accessibility to drugs, alcohol and material goods to their advantage (or disadvantage), must not engage in thievery, inebriation and addictive behavior; must be free of drugs and scrupulously honest. By the very nature of her profession and the history thereof the nurse has a very difficult task to accomplish. She has to be willing to be supervised by her peers, by a hierarchy of her colleagues, by the physicians who are her "bosses." She has to be a role model for those she serves, for her colleagues and for those who come after her. Thus, succinctly stated, the nurse's lot is not an easy nor an independent one!

In summary this chapter describes those nurses who chose a profession which required not only knowledge, ability to face difficult life and death situations; a need for meticulousness and honesty, a need to follow instructions, to be able to lead and to accept leadership; to be flexible yet steadfast; to have many attributes that they could not fulfill. They are the small minority who for many reasons that cannot be easily explained gave in to their temptations. Their background, their upbringing, their feelings of deprivation, their attitude, their ethics or lack of same, all may have played a part in their unacceptable behavior. They may have had expectations that did not materialize and possibly were consciously or unconsciously acting out their losses from an earlier period in their lives. They may have had the compulsive behavior to take, to give to themselves for feelings of inadequacy and inner deprivations. There are innumerable reasons for the behaviors of the individuals described but ultimately the public cannot afford to continue them in the caring profession of nursing!

It must be stressed again that although all of the cases here cited are authentic ones but their names, the places where they lived and practiced have all been changed to protect their identity and those of others who live and work in the places described.

Chapter V
The More Vulnerable Ones

In this Chapter we must once again remind the reader that the actions and behaviors of nurses here described are those of a small minority. The majority of nurses are honest, caring and trustworthy people who want to help humanity and who want to assist in the betterment and health of the patients they serve. They diligently work hard toward that end and they are sincerely striving to make this world a healthier and better place in which to live.

An average of 195,000 people in the United States died due to potentially preventable in-hospital medical errors in each of the years two thousand, two thousand one and two thousand and two. Associated with these errors was a cost of more than six billion dollars per year, according to a study of thirty seven million patients records that were released by Health Grades, "the health care quality company." The errors include errors made by physicians, pharmacists, nurses and other health care personnel. They include surgical mistakes such as amputations of the wrong limb; giving the wrong type of blood to patients needing transfusions, overdosing or incorrect medications given, or needed, medications not given. With greater vigilance most of the errors that have here been cited could have been avoided. There is little evidence that patient safety has improved in the last five years. "The equivalent of three hundred ninety jumbo jets full of people are dying each year due to likely preventable, in- hospital errors." These errors do not include the medical or medication errors made in nursing home facilities in this country. In these facilities it is the medication nurse who medicates the vulnerable, frail residents who are the unfortunate victims of these deadly mistakes.

The relationship between nurse and patient is a very important aspect of nursing. It is true in all settings where nursing takes place. In some institutions nurses find it difficult to exhibit and practice this caring, giving and demanding profession. It is unfortunate that sometimes the least stable nurses enter the areas which require the most and the best from the staff. Prisons are such places. They have a tendency to attract the least caring, the least ambitious and those who lack the stability that is necessary in the health care professional. They emotionally mirror the distrust, the attitude and the anger of the prison inmates. They do not take their charges seriously, are aware that these folks have lost their civil rights and have learned that their voices are, for the most part, ignored. If the inmates do complain there is no one who takes them seriously so that their physical and psychic wounds are covered with the proverbial band-aid.

It has been observed that the prison nurse is for the most part fearful when giving care to a prisoner. Fear of violence and other misconduct are very much a part of the feelings exhibited by the care giver. This can lead to the giving of inadequate, flawed or non existent healthcare as well as lack of attention to the helpless, who are in need of such care.

In order to be assured of a measure of safety the nurse takes a guard into the cell with her. He is there to protect her from any altercation that could occur and that might menace or injure the nurse in question. If she is disliked by the guards of the institution they will not accompany her nor will they lend protection to her. Therefore she must be in the guards good graces lest she be exposed to possible injury. The prisoner too is extremely vulnerable since his complaints are not given credence, his pain is rarely considered important nor is it taken seriously.

It has been frequently noted that the prison nurse is not one who over extends herself or works too hard.. Aside from the fear, at times she also has to tend to some serious wounds which take her immediate attention.

It must be noted here that there are some nurses who can find no work near their home except for an opening in a prison in their immediate vicinity. Another reason why some nurses take such a prison job is inexperience, good intentions toward the inmates and higher salaries than elsewhere. Again it must be stressed that the majority of nurses are well meaning and honest professionals who have a strong desire to serve humanity, to have a little prestige and to contribute to society by serving in the very important field of nursing.. Prisoners are a population who are desperately in need of quality health care. It is therefore unfortunate that the conditions as they stand today in prisons are not conducive to a better environment in which to furnish such care to a segment of humanity who are so much in need.

The prison nurse does have to make some difficult decisions since a medical doctor does not live on the premises of the prison. He may not be immediately available, thus it is up to the nurse to determine the course of action. It does happen that a fracas occurs in which one or more prisoners are injured. If the injury was caused by the guards and the nurse makes the physician aware of this she is in jeopardy with the guard staff and the outcome may make her very vulnerable should she need assistance from them at a future time. If she does not make a report of an incidence as mentioned, she is considered unethical and her license and her professional standing may be in danger. This places her in a "push/pull" situation, because she cannot do both at the same time. That puts her in a very vulnerable position. Two such cases have been cited in an earlier chapter:

A seriously emotionally disturbed prisoner was attacked by another inmate. The inmate ridiculed the sick individual who was saying some irrational phrases in a repetitious fashion. Being an obsessive person the man in question was unable to cease his irrational outpourings. The angry fighting inmate became entangled with the "babbler" and punched him a few times screaming "shut up." Along came two large hostile guards, separated the two men and beat the sick prisoner repeatedly into his stomach, into his head, below the belt until this man fell to the ground. They then dragged him mercilessly along the floor, thumping the man's head repeatedly. The prisoner was bleeding profusely and his eyes rolled in his head. In this condition he was dragged to the nurse's small room. Before she took his pulse and listened to his chest she had a conversation with the guards who advised her to "leave that crazy chump alone." Within the hour of this occurrence and before the nurse called an ambulance this prisoner was dead!

Another incident

involved a woman who was in the end stages of her pregnancy in a cell when she had severe pains in her abdomen. She screamed for help but was ignored. She was told by a female guard that she was not ready to deliver since she was not yet in her ninth month. (The woman herself was not certain exactly when she had conceived but she believed it was eight months earlier). The aide ultimately informed the nurse concerning this patient but found her asleep in her cubicle. When she was awakened this nurse shouted: "Let that dumb fucked up slut wait, maybe it will teach her a little lesson together with that no good bastard inside of her." When the nurse finally arrived at the cell of the prisoner several hours later, the woman was in agony, writhing and screaming in pain. She had massive vaginal bleeding, had experienced severe labor pains, but could not deliver the baby. Ultimately the infant ceased moving, the heart had stopped, the fetus had died within her mother's womb.

Clara Jamison studied for her RN degree after she had raised her three children. She and her husband lived on a farm near a small town. The nearest hospital was a considerable distance from their family home. There was little opportunity for jobs in the vicinity. Clara did discover a position for a registered nurse in the maximum security prison which was within six miles of the Jamison house. Clara applied and was accepted. She eagerly took the position and honestly believed that she could help the prisoners who would be in her care. She came to the place with much enthusiasm and energy. The prisoners seemed to like her and did not hesitate to request her help whenever they were ill or felt pain both physically and emotionally. She was very accommodating and showed a great deal of empathy and caring. The days were not long enough to handle the many requests that were made of her. It did not take too many weeks before the guards informed her that she was being too solicitous to her charges and that they were too busy to enter the cells with her as requested. They belittled the efforts that she put into her work. She especially noticed the antagonism of one of the guards toward a prisoner. Whenever this man would request to see the nurse the guard was exceptionally slow in approaching Nurse Clara on the prisoner's behalf. This attitude caused antagonism between the guard, Clara and the prisoner(Anton). There came a time when the guard completely ignored Anton. The latter was in extreme pain when he made a request for medication to relieve abdominal pain. Ultimately Nurse Clara passed by Anton's cell and heard him screaming and writhing in pain. She approached a guard who reluctantly accompanied Clara into the cell.

> She examined him and soon thereafter telephoned the physician in charge. He concurred with her decision that Anton needed to be sent to the hospital with possible appendicitis. By the time this man was admitted to the hospital he was very ill since his appendix had ruptured. Fortunately he survived. This incident and a number of other problems convinced Clara that she could not function effectively in the setting in which she found herself. She fully realized that if she did not cater to the guards she could not serve in an honest nursing capacity.

> Subsequently she was brought up before the nurse board because an accusation was leveled against her by the relatives of a victim of negligence. She was not responsible for the occurrence since she had not been notified in a timely manner of the patient's condition, nor of the fact that he was in need of immediate attention. She ultimately left her job as prison nurse!

In addition to prisoners, another very vulnerable population are the elderly in hospitals and nursing facilities. The aged are considered the undesirables by the medical establishment. The care given to younger people far exceeds the quality extended to the old. They are for the most part not acutely ill and cures are not readily found for them. There are a number of reasons for the dislike of the aged. There is the concept of gerontophobia: The fear and hatred of the old. People do not like identifying with that age group since they see themselves as getting old and don't want to admit that this too will someday be their fate. Health care staff feel these folks are not curable with their multitude of infirmities. They do not wish to form relationships with the very old since they know these peoples' years are numbered. Therefore, unless money is to be had from them few want to get involved. Many people also feel that the old have too many needs and too many requests. The caregivers have neither the time, nor the energy to satisfy the geriatric patients. They are not kept in hospitals very long and are transferred to "rehabilitation" centers and/or nursing homes to make space for the young, more acute cases. Money is one of the major roots of such actions.

It is furthermore believed that the old are too close to the grave to see substantial results from care provided for them. Thus the elderly feel hopeless and helpless and reluctantly accept the role of victim and the treatment that they receive. As a group the poor or middle class old are considered "non – persons." They are ignored and patronized regardless of their past status or accomplishments (unless of course they are wealthy or famous).

The facts concerning health care for the old are these: While old Americans are over twelve percent of our population, they use about one third of our health care expenditures every year. This discrepancy has been used to propose that Medicare limit the amount an old person may receive; that insurance companies put a lid on payments for the old; that the old be categorically excluded from hospitals and doctors' offices.

> Steffan Klauss, a very thoughtful septuagenarian, insisted that he had lived too long. He felt that he was a burden to his family and society since he was using a great deal of medication for his various physical problems, none of them however seemed to be of major proportions, nor would they have caused his death. He became so depressed that he stopped eating, drank very little water or other liquids and died a slow agonizing death by his own hands. Richard Lamm the erstwhile governor of Colorado made the statement that "the old have a duty to die and get out of the way," thus inviting the unwanted old to commit suicide

Nurses become the unlicensed physicians in nursing homes since physicians seldom visit their patients except very perfunctorily. When the doctors do visit they don't take the patients complaints seriously. Instead they pat them on the head or shoulder and tell them that "it takes time to feel better." They joke about the constipation problems from which so many of the aged suffer, but they do dictate into the patients records as is stipulated by the State Health Department. They also prescribe medication for patients, frequently by telephone, at the request of the nurse. Thorough examinations in nursing homes are almost non existent. Physicians generally believe that the patient is in the nursing home to die anyway and that therefore there is no point in wasting valuable time on a very ill, very old, impoverished patient. If the nursing staff does not promptly notify the physician of a patient's death, he does not become aware of this but nevertheless writes into the patients chart as if he had personally, on the site, confirmed the death.

Because of the great responsibility that the nurse has in nursing homes, she also has the burden and responsibility when errors and patient harm occurs.

Charles Kent an eighty three year old man was taken to the hospital because he was very weak, had difficulty eating and had swelling in his arms and legs. He was assigned a physician because his primary care doctor was not admitted to the hospital in which he found himself, (nor did he seem interested in this patient to any great extent). Charles wife, a frail octogenarian, was driven to the hospital by a friend to see her spouse to whom she had been married for more than fifty years. Mr. and Mrs. Kent were childless and thus they had no one to advocate for them, other than their elderly friend. Mrs. Kent wanted to know the diagnosis of her spouse but none of the hospital personnel answered this very reticent woman's questions. She asked for the name of the assigned physician and left several notes for him about her concerns. There was no response from him. After seven days in the hospital Charles Kent was assigned to a nursing home which was a considerable distance from this couple's home. He was in that place for two days when he became very ill, dehydrated so that his ability to consume food decreased. He was returned to the hospital where very little was done for him. It was obvious that he could not feed himself, yet a large serving of chicken and various accompaniments were set before him. When Mrs. Kent asked some questions of the nurse she claimed she could not tell her anything and the privacy law "HIPAA" precluded her from answering questions about the man's condition. She asked again to see his physician but still there was no answer from the "healer" regarding his treatment or his diagnosis. A few days later the man died. His final diagnoses were those of kidney and heart failure.

It is again obvious that no one took responsibility for this patient or his wife's concerns. For the most part they were ignored by their health care providers.

Residents in nursing facilities, especially those whose cognition has been affected adversely by the aging process and their illness, do not receive the care that they need. The night shift is more frequently responsible for such neglect. This is the case for a number of reasons: Between the hours of 11 p.m. and 7 a.m. the care givers are often tired from a busy day and have not enough opportunity for sleep. (Again we must remind our readers that most nurses are responsible professionals who carry out their duties effectively). They may choose the night shift because they have children at home and they need to be available to them during day time hours; they may resent supervision and are able to be more self sufficient or more lax when patients are asleep. They may feel that the work is not as strenuous as it is the other three shifts and they can be more relaxed. They may have greater opportunities to find a night job because of the undesirability of the "graveyard shift." Being in need of money they may choose the night work in order to earn the bonus increment for accepting the late hours. Some nurses attempt to work more than one job in order to increase their financial stability. For a number of reasons here discussed as well as a number of other reasons not defined here the old face many problems.

> Jane Randolph, LPN, mother of three, accepted a job at Manor Haven, a two hundred bed geriatric facility in a small town She was assigned the night shift since she was given a higher hourly wage than

she would have received during the other two shifts. After tending to her children all day she generally came to work exhausted. She seemed to push herself hard to keep from falling asleep. Her responsibilities were on the wing with the most needy residents. There was much crying out at night since these folks were often in pain, didn't know day from night and wanted much attention. There were two "wanderers" who were to be closely monitored since they were unsteady and were prone to falls. One, a Larry Jackson was exceptionally active one night. Nurse Jane decided to restrain him tightly into his wheel chair and left him in his room. She told the aide to take care of the other residents and that she would oversee Mr. Jackson. She closed the door of Larry's room and ignored him the remainder of the night. She was able to ignore his now muffled screams and was relieved when they stopped. At six thirty a.m she opened the door of Larry's room and found him upside down, wheelchair on top of him in an unconscious state. With the assistance of an aide she managed to untangle his restraint but he was unarousable. This man's life threatening injuries were the result of neglect by a nurse who was tired, unprofessional in her attitude and actions, who did not follow the tenets of her profession.

Neglect of the patient, especially the vulnerable elderly has been known to occur because the caregiver nurse is a heavy drug user. That includes the nurse addicted to alcohol or mind altering medication. Since the nurse has access to the narcotics cabinet it is not too difficult to divert medication.

Antonia Babbitt, RN, night supervisor in Rest Haven had worked in the Haven for three years. She was in the habit of sleeping soundly during her break and was known to oversleep her allotted time off. There was not much commotion around this issue since the other staff members had more freedom when Antonia was out of sight. When Antonia did not appear exhausted or with a glazed expression she could become very caustic with her supervisees. On a midnight shift in late December the Licensed Practical Nurse who was passing medications found a shortage of Demerol. When she looked for her supervisor she found Antonia semi responsive and incoherent. The LPN needed this medication for a terminally ill seventy nine year old male patient who was in excruciating pain. He desperately needed relief but his prescribed dosage was missing along with other pain reducing drugs that had been stored in the narcotics closet.

Antonia was taken to the emergency room of a nearby hospital and it was discovered that she was "inebriated." A report was subsequently made to the Director of Nursing and ultimately Ms. Babbitt was terminated by the Rest Haven. A report was made to the State Board of Nursing and the proceedings for a disciplinary hearing were begun. Ms B. refused to accept entering a drug rehabilitation program which would have meant giving up her license for a time to determine whether rehabilitation could be instituted here.

In examining this woman's background it was found that she had a difficult childhood. Her father was in a maximum security prison for burglary and assault. He had been incarcerated from the time that Antonia was six years old. Her mother was an inadequate care giver who had five children by several men. She was an alcoholic and Antonia, as the second oldest child was frequently left to her own devices and was expected to help the younger children to whatever food was available in the un-stocked refrigerator. Antonia was a very good student despite her deprived childhood. She was placed in a foster home as a teen, went to a middle class school and did very well. She was ambitious and was determined to do a better job than her own mother had done. She decided to be a nurse, wanted to be helpful to people in need and at the same time to be loved for the help she could extend. She took a nursing course in high school and with government help continued her education and did very well in her studies. She passed the State Board examination and received her RN license. For some time she enjoyed her work and succeeded on her job. She was pleased having a regular income and being able to afford the essentials and a few of the luxuries that were often missing as she was growing up. She never totally felt a part of the other nurses with whom she worked. Even though a number of patients treated her with gratitude and a degree of deference she often felt depleted and used. It worsened as time went by. When a patient became too demanding she became depleted and subsequently angry. When she felt exploited she would become harsh, taking on the evil, punishing mother role that she had experienced in her childhood. As time went by she discovered that she was able to relax if she medicated herself with narcotics. It did not take long before she was addicted and was able to drown out the feeling of inadequacy that was plaguing her. What she had disliked most during her childhood, her alcoholic addicted mother's behavior, had become her own.

Dimaura Kaban, was employed at the West Side Nursing Center as a certified nurse' assistant for three years after graduating from high school. She liked her work with the patients, was friendly and kept them clean and fed. She very much wanted to be a nurse even while she was in St. Thomas, the place where she grew up. Since there were not many opportunities for her in the place of her birth, she decided to immigrate to the United States to seek work and get her post high school education. She was admitted to a community college and after two years of training she received her nursing degree. Although she had a little problem with her licensing examination she passed after the second try and received her diploma as a licensed practical nurse.

Having known Dimaura as an aide, West Side continued to employ her and changed her status to LPN following the successful completion of her nursing licensing examination. Dimaura was very proud and happy to enter the profession that she had struggled long and hard to attain.

> Although Ms. Kaban had gotten along well with the nursing and other staff in her position as aide, the situation seemed to change when she received her new credentials. She felt ostracized and ignored both by the nurses and her former aide employee colleagues. She believed that the nursing supervisors were "bossing" her too much and the friends from the aide personnel pool were jealous of her and were watching her closely. She sounded almost paranoid in expressing these feelings.

Dimaura seemed to have lost the positive feelings that she had exhibited prior to her promotion. She was somewhat surly to the patients and resented their relatives when they came to visit. Because she was of the black race she felt discriminated against and did not hide her attitude in voicing her beliefs. When it was pointed out to her that many of her colleagues were also of her race she refused to recognize the connection. She seemed to be angry much of the time that she was on duty and if her assistance was needed to help one of the aides or nurses she responded grudgingly. Her former age mates and colleagues felt it difficult being around Dimaura for the past few months that she had been employed in her new capacity.

After eight months as an LPN there were a number of occurrences that ultimately brought this young woman to the attention of the Nurse Board. She had been given ample opportunities to learn the tasks that were necessary to be a competent practitioner. She had several weeks of orientation including in service training in both physical and psychological aspects of her job. She verbally assured her supervisor of her competence and her abilities to be an effective team member and nurse of the West Side Nursing Facility.

The charges that were brought against her were as follows:

First – Professional misconduct. Negligence on more than one occasion:

On December 3, 2003 while employed as a licensed practical nurse at the West Side Nursing Facility the Respondent failed to administer Procell protein supplement to an 89 year old patient ,T.R., at four p.m. as ordered by her physician.

On or about December 3 Respondent packed 78 year old patient L.L.'s wound with dry sterile gauze pads rather than Kaltostat as ordered by the physician.

On or about December 4, 2003 Respondent flushed 92 year old patient's feeding tube with 60 cc of saline rather than 150 cc of saline as ordered by the physician.

On or about December 5, 2003 Respondent administered seventy five cc of FiberSource to patient PH rather than 150 cc as ordered by the physician.

On or about December 6 Respondent failed to administer prednisone 10 mg and selan and zinc cream to patient D.M. as ordered by the physician.

Second – Specification of Professional Misconduct:

Respondent is charged with committing professional misconduct in that Respondent failed to administer Procell to 89 year old patient, T.R. at 4 p.m as ordered by the physician.

The Respondent had most recently been in an altercation with the family of a sick patient who needed to be fed. The patient's lunch had arrived at noon and the nurse needed to take care of this woman. Instead of getting the patient started (because of the danger of choking the nurse had to supervise the feeding) she ran out of the room shouting at the woman's daughter that she, the nurse, was hungry also and the patient should wait until she would be finished with her lunch and "not one minute before." This was so upsetting that the family reported this incident to the nursing supervisor. There had been several family members in the room during this occurrence who witnessed this scene.

In reviewing LPN Kaban's situation the following history of the beginning of her employment situation was discussed. At the time she began to practice nursing at West Side Nursing Facility her manager and supervisor felt that she needed to have an extended orientation period, related to passing medication,giving treatment an d learning required documentation. This was done and Dimaura spent an additional two weeks on orientation to fine tune her practice and better understand her role. Between this time and the time the initial disciplinary action was taken, her nurse manager and her supervisor, both registered nurses had several conversations with her regarding accurate documentation to ensure that all medications were given as ordered by the patients physicians.

On December 8 Dimaura Kaban, LPN received a verbal warning related to performance issues, specifically in relation to passing medication and administration of treatments. It was also related to Dimaura that she can not sign for tasks that she has not actually done, as this was falsification of documents. She was strongly encouraged to ask questions of her supervisor if she was unsure of a medication or treatment. She was asked if she felt she needed additional orientation or training and if she would like to have another nurse to work with her one on one to assist with time management and organization. She promptly declined these suggestions. She was asked what the nursing facility team could do to facilitate her performance and she stated that she could think of nothing. She posed no questions.

Later in December the evening supervisor spent three evening shifts with Dimaura, providing one on one oversight and assistance. The Supervisor on those evening shifts did not identify any overt safety issues at that time.

On December 30, a medication error and a treatment error occurred. The next day the RN supervisor prepared and subsequently gave Ms. Kaban, LPN a warning. She had not administered Procell as ordered as directed by the physician, but signed the medication sheet as if she had done this. The treatment error was significant, as it was for a resident with a stage four sacral decubitus ulcer. Dimaura did not follow the physician's orders, which were clearly stated.. In addition, this written warning again restated that there were multiple omissions of signatures by this LPN on the medical sheets, despite numerous interactions with the nurse manager and supervisor, as well as having had a previous verbal warning. A day later, Dimaura wrote her version of events and submitted it. She stated in her rebuttal that in regard to the treatment error, that she had followed what another nurse had told her to do "which means to disregard whatever the treatment order was in the book." She had also documented that the "allegations made were false," therefore she insisted that she was wrongly and maliciously accused.

There was another meeting with the respondent Dimaura and her relief charge nurse, "N.M." LPN, that week, and the issues were discussed once again. Dimaura acknowledged that she had disregarded the physician's orders for this treatment as she "didn't want to make the other nurse mad," so she did not follow the orders. (the "other nurse" was the one who had reported the condition of the patient's decubitus the previous day.)LPN Dimaura stated that she did not check the medical record to review the actual physician's order for this treatment, nor did she contact the supervisor for clarification. Much time was spent with Dimaura on that particular afternoon to attempt to get her to comprehend the severity of not following doctor's orders and signing for tasks that were not done. She was told that these were issues that could potentially affect the status of her license and that the Office of Professional Discipline of the State may become involved if these issues were not resolved immediately. Ms.

Kaban was again offered additional assistance but she declined, stating that "she understood."

The next day significant issues regarding the nursing practices by Dimaura Kaban occurred. A written report from the nurse manager was sent to the Director of Nursing re. an altercation which had occurred between LPN Kaban and a patient's family. The daughter of said patient approached the Nurse and asked her to start her father's tube feeding. This family member, who is also a nurse, stated that Dimaura only gave one third of the flush to her father, not the full amount as ordered. When Ms. Kaban ignored the request the patient's daughter approached another nurse to intervene to ensure that her father receive the appropriate care. The other nurse provided the additional fluid requirement for this resident as well as administered his medications which were also several hours late. (The nurse who now had assisted in correcting the flushing was the evening supervisor who had alleged at another time that she had found no problem during the three previous shifts when she had been asked to observe and assist Dimaura). When this family member asked Dimaura about only giving fifty cc vs. l50cc, the LPN reportedly stated: "If you want him to have more water, you'll have to get it yourself," and gestured toward the bathroom. The tube feeding rate of administration was set incorrectly as well. Dimaura had received one on one instruction on how to set the pumps the day before all this took place. It was furthermore reported by this patient's daughter that Dimaura had spilled a large amount of tube feeding on this resident's floor and left it there. The resident's daughter cleaned it herself with towels.A final written warning was prepared related to the above issues and was presented to Ms. Kaban by the nurse manager. All issues were reviewed with her. At this time, her practice was sanctioned and she was removed from the evening shift. She was mandated to the day shift where she would be closely observed on a one on one basis by another nurse for at least six day shifts over a two week period. Problems would be addressed immediately by observing the nurse for obvious safety issues. If the issues were not resolved during this time and improvement to standard not noted or sustained, she would be terminated. This was made very clear to Dimaura and she was in agreement to the mandates which were presented to her. The State's Office of Professional Discipline was notified that Dimaura Kaban's practice was being sanctioned. The Nurse was informed that this sanction was reported to the regulatory agency.

Dimaura was observed three times on three different day shifts. A multitude of potentially significant errors would have occurred if she had not had oversight by another professional. She was unable to complete medication pass within allotted time frames for all three morning medication passes, which resulted in the supervising nurse taking over for her. Multiple times, medications would have been omitted, an entire page of medications was missed for one resident, an extra dose of a medication was pulled for one resident, an antidepressant was pulled for administration but was forgotten and she did not know how to use ACE wraps to bilateral lower extremities for one resident. In addition she opened the incorrect resident's drawer and began to pull medications for the wrong resident. When preparing to do the treatment for the resident mentioned above with the Stage four decubitis, Dimaura asked the supervising nurse what an intercath is...this treatment has not changed and an intercath had been used for an extended period of time for flushing the wound. The evening shift supervisor had shown Dimaura what the intercath was and how to use it months ago when she demonstrated the treatment on this patient. Following the treatment, Dimaura had left soiled towels in the garbage can of this resident's room. These towels were used in the wound irrigation process on this resident and had become contaminated with bodily fluids, illustrating significant lack of infection control practices. Ms. Kaban's final observed medication pass occurred a day later. Documentation of the observations were submitted and discussions were initiated with the two nurse managers, the head of Human Resources and the Director of Nursing and the decision to terminate Dimaura's employment immediately was clear.

The Nurse Manager and the Director of Nursing subsequently met with Dimaura and the concerns of the Facility were reviewed with her and the results of the observations were shared with her. As a result Dimaura Kaban was justifiably terminated from her position at West Side Health Facility. This woman did not understand the magnitude of her area of deficiency, and felt that she had done everything correctly during the observations, even though she required frequent intervention by the supervising nurses. Even when she was given specific examples, provided supplemental information regarding her performance and potentially negligent practice , she still did not agree that she had performed at a less than desirable standard. She was told that the Office of Professional Discipline was involved and that they were being called to inform them of her termination of employment.

She adamantly refused to sign her termination notice, but left the facility without incident.

In examining this situation one must wonder how this person graduated from a nursing school, how she passed the licensing examination and in view of her alleged past learnings did she not know some of the must rudimentary knowledge that is necessary in carrying out adequate nursing duties. How could she have escaped, for example, the very stringent rule of infection control, chart recording, medication pass and the essential nature of giving the prescribed medications correctly.

In nursing homes the staff deals with the most vulnerable adult patients who cannot defend themselves and need protection. This population consists of patients/residents who are for the most part incapable of taking care of themselves. They often feel degraded and alone; they are frail, most likely in their eighties, have limited financial, emotional and mental resources; their hearing and eyesight are likely to be diminished. They are the folks who depend on the staff, especially the nursing staff, to treat them kindly, with compassion and very importantly to see that their health care is handled with precision and cautious care in order to give them the maximum health possible under their particular circumstances.

> Sharon Drake, RN was a very attractive young nurse who enjoyed having "a good time." She was friendly with the staff of Greenfield Manor where she worked a twelve hour shift three nights per week. She seemed to like the very frail elderly patients and they would look forward to her time at the institution. She would make them smile and for a little while they were able to forget their pain. She was very gentle and understanding and responsive to their needs. There was a rumor that Ms. Drake enjoyed being the life of whatever party she attended, but it did not seem to affect her work. One night Sharon was substitute supervisor of the unit in which she worked. Since the "medicine" nurse had the evening off Ms. Drake also passed out the medications. She seemed unusually talkative and it was noted by several staff members that on the night of November 21, 2002 she was somewhat unsteady and an odor of alcohol was detected.

She did manage to distribute the medications to her assigned charges and afterwards retreated to the nursing office, turned out the lights and fell asleep. When one of the aides needed her she was difficult to arouse. There was a problem with several of the patients. She had given the wrong medication to these folks as well as documenting these medications in other patient's charts. Since she was well liked the other staff members had their doubts about her condition but chose not to report what they believed had taken place. The one aide, whose grandmother was a patient was concerned and made mention of the fact that "there seemed to be something wrong" with Nurse Sharon. When questioned by the Director of Nursing about the previous night's occurrence Ms. Drake denied any wrong doing. The aide who had reported Sharon retracted her statement, alleging that she might have been mistaken in what she surmised. It was not long after this incident that a quantity of the narcotic Demerol was missing repeatedly over a number of days. It was discovered that RN Drake had diverted this drug for her own use. She succeeded in this endeavor in the following fashion: The Respondent (nurse Sharon) with fraudulent intent, documented in the Medical Surgical Division's narcotic "record of dispensing," that the controlled drug, Demerol, was administered to patient "D.M." when in truth and in fact, as the Respondent well knew, it was not. A day after this event Nurse Sharon with fraudulent intent documented in the Medical Surgical Divison's narcotic record that the controlled drug Demerol was administered to patient "CK." When in truth and in fact, as the Respondent well knew, it was not. These actions were repeated innumerable times. It was estimated that she did this too many times before her fraudulent deeds were uncovered. Unfortunately it took many months before proof of this woman's diversions were uncovered and she was subsequently terminated from her job. The State's Nurse Board was notified by the administration of the Nursing Facility.

A number of hearings before a nurse board were scheduled with this Nurse, witnesses for and against the respondent appeared. At first there was much denial on Sharon's part. She had employed an attorney to defend her actions. The witnesses who spoke in her behalf described her as a woman of "good" moral character, helpful, friendly, generous to a fault and unassuming. Her accusers were staff from the nursing facility where the fraudulence occurred and two relatives of patients who had seen their loved ones in pain without the medication that was prescribed for them. At the conclusion of the hearings the ultimate outcome was that Ms, Drake was guilty as charged. She was an addict, a drug user and the recommendation of the Nurse Board's jury panel was unanimous. A disciplinary penalty was exacted upon the respondent and upon her license as well as her registration, which had been previously granted to the Respondent to practice as a licensed registered nurse.

When examining the background of Ms. Drake it was found that she was from a fairly large family whose father was an alcoholic and whose mother was addicted to a number of medications. Both parents seemed to have been anesthesising themselves from the vagaries of life. The mother a hypochondriac, always wanted her daughter to become a nurse to help with her various maladies. Sharon complied with her mother's wishes but at times felt her nursing duties to be somewhat overwhelming . In the beginning of her career she was very proud and happy to have succeeded in that endeavor. She found working with the geriatric patients rewarding since they often praised her and responded positively to her winning smile. At other times she found the pressures to answer the patients multitudinous needs and wants difficult. It was during those times that she turned to alcohol and later to drugs. The narcotics were accessible to her and she was certain that her theft would go unnoticed. It seemed so easy to drown her pain by these means. Even though she had witnessed the occasional alcoholic stupors that her father was in and the ingesting of her mother's many pain killers, she did not directly identify her deviant actions and behaviors with theirs. It was only after her hard earned license was revoked that she fully realized the seriousness of her situation and what she had done to herself.

There are times when nurses become the vulnerable ones. There have been a number of cases in which innocent nurses were accused of wrong doing without any cause. In addition there are situations in which a very minor and human occurrence takes place which is misinterpreted with greater concern than it deserves. Two such authentic incidents will here be cited:

Emily Grande, RN had worked in a small hospital for sixteen years and was well thought of by the physicians, the patients she cared for and the community in which she lived. She was always willing to give advice or assistance to a neighbor or friend who had a health problem and would go the proverbial extra mile to give the best care within her capabilities. She was conscientious, always on time, had nothing negative in her personnel record and had received a number of excellent evaluations for the years that she had been an employee of the hospital. She was supervising nurse on the night shift. It was at midnight, after she had worked an additional three hours to cover for a nurse who could not be there on time that night, that she had severe pain in her arm and shoulder. She would ordinarily have been able to go home to take care of herself but there was no one available on her shift to cover the necessary time. She helped herself to two Motrin tablets which she swallowed with a glass of water to relieve her excrutiating pain and to enable her to finish caring for her patients until relief would come.

One of the Aides observed her taking these tablets and reported her to the Director of Nursing. The medication taken was removed from a blister pack which had belonged to a patient who had been discharged. The rule of the hospital was that medication is supposed to be removed from a medicine cart and placed into a discontinued box when a patient leaves or when a physician discontinues a medication. The pharmacist or an employee of the drug store comes once a month to pick it up, and the excess medicine is reported back to the insurance company and credited back to the patient's account. There was much discussion around this situation and when Nurse Emily was brought before the disciplinary board she was charged as being guilty, by a preponderance of the evidence, violating the specification of professional misconduct. She was further charged with practicing the profession of nursing fraudulently. In this context fraud consists of misrepresentation or concealment in regard to some fact or material to a transaction that is made with knowledge of its falsity and with the intent to deceive another.

The jury panel unanimously recommended the nurse receive a Censure and Reprimand; be fined five hundred dollars and be placed on probation for six months. She furthermore would have to attend and complete an ethics course.

When investigating this case it was learned that the Aide who reported Nurse Emily disliked her and was able to get revenge by reporting her. She felt that Ms. Grande was domineering and viewed her, the Aide, with disdain.

The punishment seems far in excess of this so called "crime." For most folks it would hardly be worthy of a "slap on the hand." It is seriously doubtful whether any one under normal circumstances would have accused this woman of fraud.

Jean Reardon, a registered nurse was falsely accused of fraudulence by a woman, Elisa J. who was her patient. Ms. Reardon graduated from a well known psychiatric hospital with a Bachelors degree in Nursing. She then received a Master's degree in nursing and a doctorate in nursing, five years later. She attended an excellent Institute of Psychological Studies for a post-doctoral program. Doctor Reardon is a clinical nurse specialist in adult psychiatric mental health nursing and conducts a private practice in psychotherapy.

The accusations made against Jean Reardon were as follows: Verbal abuse during sessions with the complainant and insisted the complainant continue the medication Prozac when the medical doctor had discontinued it; may have improperly represented herself to secure insurance reimbursement; wrote untruths in the complainant's record.

When Dr. Reardon, RN was asked how she came to know the complainant, she explained that an insurance company of which she is a provider had directed this patient to her for psychotherapy. The insurance person had asked Dr. Reardon at the time of the referral whether she felt she could possibly take care of Mrs. J., a very problematic patient who had difficulty in the past with other therapists. Dr. Reardon agreed to take her on as a patient since she had experience with other difficult patients who had been a challenge. It was shortly thereafter that Ms. J. became Dr. Reardon's patient. It was after many months of treatment that Elisa J. apparently called the insurance company and spoke with an insurance physician and complained about the therapist. (The insurance companies do audit records and take note of patient complaints). The insurance physician telephoned the therapist to discuss this woman's allegations against her. After fifty sessions the problems began. The mutual goals that the therapist and the patient had were to work through the conflicts and anxieties of the patient and to help her learn to trust her therapist and others and to cope more effectively and to lessen her stress and anxiety.

Dr. Reardon had to telephone the insurance company, to report progress and to extend sessions after each set of ten sessions. The insurance company also wanted to have Ms. J. evaluated by a psychiatrist for possible pharmacological intervention/medication.

The psychiatrist who saw Ms. J. prescribed Prozac. It was several months later that the dosage of Prozac was increased. It was at that time that the patient developed a reaction in that she had dry mouth and stated she did not feel too well. The therapist subsequently stated that she asked Ms. J. to discuss her symptoms with the psychiatrist. This physician denied ever telling the patient she should stop taking the medication. Dr. Reardon adamantly stated that she does not have the authority to tell a patient to continue a medication as alleged by her accuser and that she had only told the patient to speak with her psychiatrist about the problems she was having with the medication. After this misunderstanding of what was said about the medication, the complainant became more angry which led to another misunderstanding about a cancellation or a change of appointment date. This precipitated the complaint made to the Office of Professional Discipline and the Nurse Board.

Another issue that Dr. Reardon wanted to clarify was that the complainant did tell her that she was suing her previous therapist, a man, because he had "falsified his records to the insurance" about what medications she was on when she really was not taking any medication. The complainant refused to identify the previous therapist or sign any consent that would allow the subject to get any records from the previous therapist.

In the complainant's letter, she wrote a number of different statements that she alleges the therapist made to her which were inappropriate. They were as follows: 1. "The apple does not fall far from the tree," which Dr. Reardon stated that she might have said, or something to that effect. She stated further that the complainant was very hostile insisting that she was a victim; , that she, the therapist was trying to make Ms. J. realize that she, too, was victimizing by what she was saying about other people in the manner in which she was speaking. She said that the complainant was abusing the subject by raising her voice and being hostile, and she was trying to show that as much as Ms. J was complaining about others, she was doing the same thing herself. 2. "Too bad you had such a toxic family, you might have amounted to something." The subject stated that she might have said "toxic family," however, she had tried during the therapy sessions to build the complainant up by making note of her accomplishments despite her surroundings. 3. "Too bad you could not be inoculated against your toxic parents." Dr. Reardon denied that she made such a statement. She declared that she was very empathetic and that she had not labeled the parents as toxic but spoke in generalities about her upbringing and the surroundings of the complainant. 4. "Do you think your late husband was a homosexual"? Dr. Reardon stated that during therapy sessions the patient described her past marriage as asexual. The subject felt that in the normal course of questioning and developing this issue a logical question in the family history would be that question. She feels that her client might have taken it out of context and just isolated that one particular question and forgot what was being discussed at that time. 5. "Be glad your accountant is interested in you because no one else is." The subject stated she never made such a statement. 6."You are like a cactus tree in the desert with thorns and all alone." Dr. Reardon explained that she was trying to make an analogy and may have used the metaphor of a cactus stating that even though there is a harsh outside, if you looked inside, it is good, which is what she saw in this patient. 7. "If there was a fork in the road between right and wrong, would you take the right one ?" The therapist stated that she did not recall making such a remark or asking such a question.

When the complainant received a copy of her records from Dr. Reardon, there were several statements in a number of the outpatient treatment records that the complainant felt were untrue and again grounds for misconduct in that they were written by the subject and were false. A review of these statements were made and are as follows:

1 – Delusions of treachery and deception, risk to self and others, substance use history positive and impaired social interaction. The complainant had a history of being a pariah in social groups and did not understand how her behavior effected others. Dr. Reardon did state that her checking "yes" to substance use history was wrong in that the patient did not have a substance abuse history.

2 – increase in suspicion, will not allow note taking, writing letters about former therapists and women in the church. Dr. R. stated that it was the complainant who told her that she was writing letters to the church about the women and to her minister about what was going on. Dr. R. thought that it was therapeutic to allow the complainant to continue writing the letters to the church and allowing her not to negate her feelings. Dr. R. was aware that the complainant did not like when she took notes during their sessions. She stated that this particular patient was not an easy one to forget and that many of the issues she remembers quite clearly.

3 – On an Outpatient Treatment Report Dr. R. wrote "jealous of women with attentive husbands and children, can't pay co-pay, requested increased visits." The subject stated that the patient had told her that she was alone and really had no family and spoke of her sister

who had a husband and attentive children, and she the patient apparently missed that kind of interpersonal relationship. The patient stated that no one paid attention to her, and through the interactions and discussions during that treatment, the subject deduced that the complainant longed for such a relationship and was jealous of women or people who had attentive people surrounding them. Dr. Reardon stated that she recalls the complainant saying that she had been a volunteer at Jerome Hospital and had left. However when the patient tried to return, they would not take her back, and from that she wrote that the complainant was rejected from that hospital program. Dr. R. furthermore recalled that the complainant had specifically requested increased visits and that she needed more time to discuss and resolve her issues.

4 – An entry made by Dr. Reardon stated the following: The patient had a "run in with travelers in Europe, road rage." The subject explained that as the patient was explaining her recent trip to Europe that no one wanted to sit with her, that was a topic that the patient wanted to discuss and work out. Dr. Reardon stated that she was worried about the patient's impulsiveness, especially when she had discussed a parking lot issue where a car had parked too close to her and there was a possibility of door damage. The Doctor also stated that she was concerned about the potential of the patient's physical anger and that is why she wrote in her chart "road rage."

After a thorough investigation by a public member of the Nurse Board who is also a PhD licensed psychologist, she felt although a little more finesse in the recordings and alleged conversations with the patient could have been utilized, there was no reason to bring the patient's Doctor before the jury panel for a disciplinary hearing. The patient as stated had been to a number of therapists, was pleased with none and was ready to accuse the most recent therapist of malpractice.

Psychotherapists on the whole are very vulnerable people since they frequently deal with very disturbed and distraught individuals. Records do not tell the entire story since they are not verbatim and contain only certain parts of conversations. Another problem is that which takes place in a psychotherapists office is between two people and there are no witnesses to the feelings and verbalizations that occur.

Summary

Looking at Webster's Dictionary we find that "vulnerable" means "capable of being physically wounded." The people described in this chapter are those who are wounded physically, emotionally or both. By reason of their status they are faced with serious consequences to their very being. We must realize that we see so many nurses who play a part in the acts described, is because of their profession and their own vulnerability on a daily basis with individuals whose frailties are critical and whose needs are great. Nurses see the very ill; they treat people who are in severe pain; they must deal with death and the dying; the expectations toward them are often unreal; they are the servants of the public, yet their prestige is relatively low. It is the physician who has the power and control and the nurse must follow orders. They have responsibilities often without the rewards. It must be remembered that the majority of nurses are capable, well meaning individuals who entered the profession of nursing because of their desire to help, to be in a field that appeals to them, to understand the human body, to assist in alleviating pain and in hopefully curing the sufferer. We have here chosen only those who for reasons described have failed to meet expectations of their role. Deviant behavior can be found in any profession not just in the field of health care of which nursing is a part.

When we examine the More Vulnerable Ones and why they become the victims of neglect and abuse we see people who are helpless because of their age, imprisonment or other conditions that place them in a position of powerlessness. They are folks in nursing homes, prisons and in situations which compromise them in many ways. Their voices are not heard, they are the invisible people. They can no longer "give" and depend on the will and actions of others. Some have been abandoned by their families, friends and society. Others are incarcerated and are unable to control their own lives. They are frequently judged and abused because they have no way out of their situation.

Several situations have been cited in this chapter of nurses who have been accused in situations where they were the victims. By their very position and closeness to the sick and the emotionally/mentally ill they become the objects of unsubstantiated accusations, therefore making their role a difficult one.

Chapter VI

Male Nurses

Men in a Female World

There is one more "deviant nurse" in the profession. That is the male nurse whose deviance consists solely of his sex.

As we will see, the sexual revolution, a social movement which reached crescendo volume in the 1960's did not only affect women. Demanding equality in the work place and promoting the right of women to earn a livelihood in such traditional male occupations as doctor and lawyer also led to the inclusion of men in traditionally female occupations such as flight attendant and nurse.[1]

Therefore men were first admitted to almost all nursing schools in the 1960's having been barred from nursing schools until then. Nevertheless, men have been involved in nursing in America since 1811 when the Bellevue Hospital in New York City organized the first and only school of nursing for men.[2]

Evidently, then, men have been in nursing for nearly two centuries. Nevertheless, the number of male nurses is not increasing. On the contrary. In 1995 10.7 percent of students in nursing programs were men but in 2003 only 8.4 percent of nursing students were male. Perhaps the only exception to this decline was the enrollment of 19 male nursing students at the University of Wisconsin/Madison where they constituted 13 percent of the 144 students admitted in 2004.[3]

The reason for the difficulties in enrolling men in nursing school is that men experience "negative sanctions" when they undertake to enter a profession traditionally female. This usually means that men who enter nursing school will be questioned by parents, friends and even other nursing students about their sexuality. Nursing students are labeled homosexuals even if that is not their inclination leading to a major effort by male nursing students to deny homosexuality. The result of this questioning is "role strain" which sociologists define as "tension when coping with the requirements of incompatible roles."[4] A major study by Egeland and Brown conducted in Oregon showed that many male nurses entered administration, psychiatric nursing and anaesthetics in order to cope with a female dominated profession. These specialties appear more congruent with the masculine sex role[5]

Nursing is often called "the caring profession" because it is commonly assumed that women who enter the profession have a "caring" personality. Men, by reason of sex have to first learn to be caring and therein lies a source of difficulty for men. The truth is of course that female nurses spend a great deal of time writing and relatively little time with patients. Therefore, the concern over whether men are or are not as caring as women is only hypothetical. The fact is that patients are mostly "on their own." Were this not the case, men would have to learn caring behavior before succeeding at nursing.

Male nurses report that they are less likely than female nurses to be the target of criticism when mistakes are made. There are even those who claim that sexism actually favors male nurses. [6]

There are about 2.7 million nurses in the U.S.A. Of these, 2.3 million are registered nurses. A registered nurse is one who has passed the national licensing examination known as the State Board Test Pool.[7] The others are practical nurses. Only 5.4 percent of these nurses are men. It appears therefore that men are unlikely to invade this female profession in great numbers. This prediction is hardly precarious since men have had the opportunity to enter nursing schools for the past forty years. [8]

An additional reason for the scarcity of male nurses is that nurses "drop out" of the nursing schools at a higher rate than is true of women. Since 1992, the rate at which men drop out of nursing school has increased.

The most common explanation for the dearth of male nurses is that the popular culture makes it unacceptable for men to enter nursing. These beliefs are perpetuated by the media which inevitably portray nurses as women unless a male nurse is defamed as a homosexual or at least "less than a man."[9]

If it is true that the United States will suffer a nurse shortage of 500,000 by 2020, then it may well be necessary to attract men into the profession by overcoming the popular view of male participation in this enterprise.

Nursing has never become more lucrative than in recent years. In 1997 female registered nurses earned an average salary of $37,400. Male nurses, then and now earned about three percent more. In 2004, the average salary for nurses has risen to $54, 574 although this average mean salary was not earned in all American hospitals.

The income of nurses can vary a good deal because the responsibilities of nurses range over such a large area of work. For example, anesthesiology nurses can earn $75, 000 a year although the average for peri-anesthesia nurses was $59,400 in 2004. Nurses in outpatient/clinic settings earned about $57, 000 in 2004.

A study of nurse salaries conducted in 2002 found that male nurses are paid more than female nurses. The survey showed that men earned roughly 12.3 percent more than women. About 8.3 percent of this excess was attributed to "the endowment effect," meaning that men were believed to be more productive than women. The other 91.7 percent were attributed to discrimination in favor of men.[10]

It is of course also true that men earn more on the average because male nurses are more often found in higher positions than female nurses. This is in part due to the higher levels of education attained by a greater proportion of men than women in nursing. More men have masters or doctoral degrees than is true of women so that men are more likely to attain supervisory positions than women. This advantage is not only the result of superior education. No doubt some men are given supervisory positions because they are men.[11]

Furthermore, women in all occupations are more likely to leave the occupation to raise children only to return later when men, who stayed on the job, have already attained more income and promotions which mothers had to sacrifice in behalf of their children.

Compared to other professions such as teaching and social work nurses earn as much or more. Therefore money or the salary structure can hardly explain the dearth of men in nursing.

In 1993, Anders surveyed the motivation of male nursing students. He reported that the primary motive for men to enter nursing was they like people and enjoyed helping others. Job availability and job security were also high on the list of motives for entering the profession as was interest in the biological sciences. The survey by Anders revealed that upon achieving the RN status men generally sought emergency room, intensive care or anesthesia settings.[12]

Male nursing students are generally older than female nurses because many men who enter nursing school have failed at a previous occupation. Upon entering the profession male nurses need to be re-socialized to accept the female point of view involving the care giving role which girls learn at a young age. Male nurses must also learn to examine women, a task neither they or their patients find comfortable. In addition, male nurses must learn to "get along" with mainly female colleagues.

Teamwork is very important in nursing. Here men may have an advantage because team work is regarded as an important male attribute in American life. Men in all occupations are likely to have been involved in team work, an attribute they can use in nursing.

Men who enter nursing must also learn to deal with constant criticism and discrimination. This criticism is not only derived from the assumption that male nurses play a female role but also that nursing is a low paying occupation. These assumptions need not be true to be effective. Therefore, male nurses exhibit a good deal of the same anxiety associated with any minority status. Gender role conflict is only one reason for these anxieties. More important is that men who enter nursing normally do not exhibit the assertiveness common to men in almost any setting . The need to be assertive is a long-standing male characteristic which is hard to overcome in so different an environment.

There are of course some men who are far less aggressive than is normally expected. Furthermore, men in nursing also encounter hostility from the working environment. This is most evident in the obstetrical area. Men are indeed a visible minority in that situation although the doctors who deliver babies are almost always men. This leads us to the inevitable conclusion that the aversion of many women to allow a male nurse to participate in the delivery of their baby has more to do with the social class of the male nurse than his competence.[13]

Another form of nursing care which has traditionally excluded men is pediatrics, i.e. the care of sick children. Male nurses tend to work in such areas as psychiatry, urology, administration and anesthesiology but not pediatrics. Studies have shown that there are gender differences in the manner in which care situations are handled. Currently, such care is likely to include the use of advanced technology. Often such technology causes a good deal of pain and suffering. This in turn causes nurses a good deal of anguish and can result in nurses becoming emotionally "stunted." The reason for this is that the attention of the nurse and the doctor is directed entirely to the diagnosis which is achieved by the use of all kinds of machines, instruments and technical equipment without seeing the suffering child or seeking any means to comfort him. Technique is everything, suffering is secondary.[14]

There are those who believe they can break the stereotype burdening male nurses. This may be achieved by first influencing high school guidance counselors in high schools across the country to talk to young men about a nursing career. This has already been tried in some high schools but failed at once because the recruitment materials were written with women in mind. The printed materials all showed women in white uniforms wearing a nurse hat and appearing "soft and fuzzy and warm" and not at all like men. To counteract these feminine images the Oregon Center for Nursing distributed a poster showing male nurses as members of the armed forces or snowboarding or dressed to ride a motorcycle.

The Oregon program also invites high school boys to enroll in a program that lets them follow male nurses in their work setting, participate in hands-on activities and thereby learn about the different opportunities in nursing. Male nurses also speak to school and community groups about nursing both in Oregon and in North Carolina.

In North Carolina all high school students must complete a senior project. That can be a program allowing seniors to complete a senior project on nursing. An effort is made to interest boys to choose nursing as their senior project.

Furthermore an effort is being made to recruit men into nursing. This is being conducted by the American Assembly for Men in Nursing. That organization seeks to encourage men of all ages to enter nursing and to make it easier for men to feel comfortable with such an occupational choice. Their 2004 convention was held in Tuscon, Arizona and promoted the theme: "Men in Nursing: Meeting a World of Health Care Needs."[15]

The American Assembly for Men in Nursing also hosts an Internet "chat room" where men can discuss their interest in the profession. This reveals that occupational segregation continues to be a principal obstacle to the acceptance of men in the nursing profession just as occupational segregation hinders women doctors and lawyers in those professions.

There are several explanations for occupational segregation. One is sex. Sex is a major determinant of status and sex role stereotypes are almost universal. Therefore sex typing of occupations has always existed in all human societies and American society is no exception. Such sex typing of occupations is not related to biological differences but rather to beliefs about men and women as supported by various cultures. Merton, a.k.a Meyer Skolnick, has shown that when a large number of workers in an occupation are of one sex it is usually a sign that the culture supports the view that this is how it should be.[16] High ranking occupations have traditionally been male in the United States and elsewhere so that the proportion of women decreases and the proportion of men increases as one approaches the top in occupations open to both sexes.[17]

Occupational segregation is by no means gone from the United States. This is easily demonstrated by looking at the type of work done mostly by women and men. No doubt the gender gap which existed before 1980 has gradually become narrower. Indeed, there are more female executives, doctors, lawyers and other female professionals than ever before in this country. Nevertheless, in 2003, 56 percent of all temporary health care workers were women and 72 percent of all part time workers were women as were almost all nurses, most social workers, large numbers of grade school teachers, nearly all secretaries and surely every dental hygienist in the country. All of these occupations are staffed predominantly by women and of these nursing has been most segregated because of its congruence with female traditional roles. During the entire twentieth century the proportion of females in nursing has varied from 93 percent to 98 percent. Yet, looking back at the nineteenth century it turns out that then, there were many men in nursing. However, as more lucrative occupations opened up in the twentieth century, men moved into these positions and left the nursing to women.[18]

Children's books depict nurses as women and doctors as men. High school students rank nursing lowest on a masculinity scale which include submissiveness, dependency, high religiosity, low economic opportunities and considerable social service interests. All of these characteristics are associated with femininity in American culture.[19]

Another reason for occupational segregation is tokenism. Tokenism exists when one social group is in the extreme minority or less than 15 percent. This is no longer true of female physicians and lawyers but it is true of male nurses. The evidence is that it is not the gender of men that affects their interaction with female nurses but their scarcity. Sociologists have discovered that there are perceptional tendencies which are associated with tokens. One of these is heightened visibility. This refers to the disproportionate share of attention given to token group members with the consequences that the behavior of men in nursing becomes a much more frequent topic of gossip than the behavior of women. For example, the names and even the personal lives of male nurses are known and topics of conversation in many hospitals even as the names of female nurses are not known. Furthermore, more patients seeking nursing assistance gravitate towards the male nurses who are so much more visible than the phalanx of female nurses. In addition, patients often referred to "my male nurse" but never to "my female nurse." Also, hospital employees generally knew the number of male nurses employed by that hospital but have no idea how many female nurses their hospital employs. A second perceptional tendency is contrast. Here the dominant group, in this case women, exaggerates the contrast between male nurses and female nurses and stress the traits that women have in common. Therefore, male nurses are usually excluded from the social network of the majority, female nurses. This is due to the topics of conversation as women are likely to discuss weddings, bridal showers, dating, finding a man, sexual issues and their menstrual cycle. Clothing and haircuts are also discussed by women as are the experience of giving birth. Male nurses are not invited to Tupperware parties and houseware parties. All this excludes men *ipso facto.* It is of course understood that men do not care for these topics or social events and find them uninteresting at best.[20]

Thirdly, assimilation refers to the stereotyping of all male nurses as if all male nurses were the same. This means that gender-specific traits are attributed to the tokens. For example, male nurses are asked by female nurses to do all the lifting or other muscle work. In many hospitals leadership roles are also assigned to men so that male nurses have a better chance at reaching a supervisory position than is true of the many women in the profession. Assimilation also refers to female nurses so that nurses will talk about "the girls" among themselves and evidently leave out male nurses. Women's reading material is also usually found in the work space of nurses, including *Good Housekeeping* and *Women's Day.*

Kanter argues that the interaction of the token group with the dominant group leads inevitably to "role entrapment" and performance pressure with detrimental results for the token minority. This contention by Kanter was not found in a study of male nurses made by Gans. That study revealed that male nurses were affected by their token status in many ways but that the effects for men were conducive and not detrimental as was found to be the situation for women. The reason for this difference is the token's master status. A master status is the most important status or set of privileges a person may have. In the case of men, it is their sex and gender. This is not true for women whose master status is their relationship to their nearest male relative such as father or husband. Therefore, men are propelled to greater attainment by a token status among women while women are debased by that status.[21]

Status characteristics include "expectation states." This means that it is expected that male status is associated with more favorable characteristics than is female status. Such a view therefore predicts that tokenism would have a different outcome for males than for females. In the case of nurses, however, the appropriateness of male nursing defeats the advantage men usually occupy so that both males and females are likely to expect men not to do well as nurses because the profession is associated with female attributes. Tokens have a lesser status than majorities. Men have a higher status than women. Therefore male nurses create a status conflict in the minds of the female majority which makes men marginal members of the profession.[22]

That marginality is emphasized by the common belief among female nurses, both married and single, that male nurses are "gay" i.e. homosexuals, whether true or not. Male nurses are also frequently taken for physicians despite the difference in apparel. Physicians either wear long coats with the imprint of M.D. or Dr. after or before their name while male nurses wear short white jackets revealing the RN on the uniform. The mistakes of tokens are also more often noticed and discussed by the dominant group than the mistakes of the majority. Mistakes by male nurses are far more often noticed than are mistakes by female nurses.

Yet another difference between male and female nurses is that male nurses do not have to play the "doctor-nurse" game. Male nurses can more easily associate with male physicians who may have as much influence on their career advancement as their female supervisors.[23]

Male and female conduct is derived from both socialization and expectations. Socialization deals with how we behave differently as men or women. Expectations refers to the fact that we expect male characteristics from men whether or not they have these characteristics . This is also true for women or members of various ethnic groups. This is also the reason why male nurses can more easily deal with male doctors who are most likely interested in football, the stock market and travel but have no interest in such female topics as baby showers, weddings, boyfriends and Tupperware parties. Therefore, the power of expectations is greater than the actual performance of tokens within the larger, dominant group.[24]

The Psychological Orientation of Male Nurses towards their Work

Some economists and feminists claim that working alongside women involves not only economic but also social and psychological costs for men. Such researchers claim that male dominated work affirms masculinity and is therefore imbued with positive cultural significance. Likewise, female dominated work is viewed less favorably than male dominated work. This devaluation of women's jobs compared to men's jobs leads to a loss of esteem for male nurses and threatens their masculine identity and their well-being. The social losses for men in women's occupations such as nursing are not replicated by women in men's occupations. A female airline pilot, surgeon or carpenter does not suffer a status loss for her participation in almost "men only" jobs. Male nurses suffer a great deal of status loss. Males in female dominated occupations experience status contradiction and even run the risk of weakening the entire patriarchal social structure. The point here is that some researchers claim that working alongside women has negative consequences for men *independent* of gender mix and job rewards.[25]

Status contradiction is related to ascribed and achieved status. Sociologists view ascribed status as that status with which anyone is born and which cannot be altered. This includes sex, race and age but can also include the social standing of the family and the religion into which we are born and which is imposed on us as children. Ascribed status then is "a social position a person receives at birth or assumes involuntarily later in life." An achieved status is one which is voluntary such as education, marriage or occupation. Occupation is, for most Americans, also their master status in that occupation conveys a great deal about income, competence and prestige. There are of course a few Americans whose master status is their name such as Rockefeller or Bush or Roosevelt.[26]

Every occupation, although achieved, carries with it an ascription derived from popular opinion. For example, it is believed that professors are intelligent even if that is not always the case. It is assumed that musicians are emotional and have a great deal of feeling even if that is not always the case. Likewise, male nurses are viewed by popular opinion as homosexuals. Homosexuality is widely discredited in the United States despite recent efforts to reverse this view. It is considered deviant and is ascribed to that five percent of American men who have "come out" and revealed their inclination. Homosexuals are the targets of *societal* deviance which differs from *situational* deviance in that it is ascribed to people because it is widely perceived, in advance and in general, and hence stigmatized. Situational deviance refers to an actual deed by a person who is therefore stigmatized. An example would be someone convicted of a crime whether guilty or not. Because male nurses are assumed to be homosexuals they are therefore penalized for that reason alone.[27]

Male nurses are suspect alone because they entered a profession traditionally female. They fail to meet the expectations normally associated with men's career choices. This then is the essence of the status contradiction male nurses face. Therefore male nurses may suffer a decline in self esteem leading male nurses to believe that compared to female nurses they have the lower social position. Our culture associates masculinity with the ability to earn a great deal of money or to master a skill or to exhibit great strength. None of these attributes are popularly associated with male nurses. Parsons has made the following comment concerning this status differential:

> . . .in a situation which strongly inhibits competition between the sexes on the same plane, the feminine glamour pattern has appeared as an offset to masculine occupational status and to its attendant symbols of prestige. ....It is perhaps significant that there is a common stereotype of physically beautiful women, expensively and elaborately dressed women with physically unattractive but rich and powerful men.[28]

Male nurses face yet another problem. It is popularly assumed that women are characteristically suited to be nurses and that men are not suited for that kind of work. This opprobrium does not affect female physicians because the level of skill and intelligence demanded of doctors is far greater than that demanded of nurses.

There are some students of mixed work settings who suggest that men working in female settings are not necessarily penalized and may even experience a higher well being. These researchers say that tokenism has more positive outcomes for men than women. In the case of male nurses this view is supported by the finding that male nurses have a more egalitarian interaction with male physicians than is true of female nurses. This would mean that male nurses enjoy an informal status advantage over female nurses. The influence of relative deprivation plays an important part in the manner in which male and female nurses view themselves. Comparisons to doctors is inevitable in the hospital environment where nurses and physicians work so closely together all the time. Nurses are therefore continuously saddled with the disadvantage which such status comparison imposes on them. Male "tokens" however, are likely to receive superior treatment from doctors and even some patients so that they can compare themselves favorably to their female co-workers. Furthermore, male nurses, like all men, enjoy privileges in the general society which are associated with being a man which is a master status.[29]

Scott J. South et al analyzed male and female workers in a federal bureaucracy and found that female dominated work settings do not threaten men's sense of well-being as much as "male cost" arguments claim. South shows that at least in his study male tokens were more favorably treated than female workers, but that men's minority status increased the frequency and quality of male-female interaction.[30]

The literature on intergroup relations has repeatedly shown that both male and female "tokens" had better interactions with the dominant group than when the sexes were more balanced. This is also true of other minority groups so that Jewish Americans felt no prejudice and seldom encountered discrimination before the arrival of millions of Jews in the U.S. after 1890.

Some writers suggest that men view female workers, i.e. women nurses as a competitive threat most when the gender mix is balanced. If that is so, then the small minority of male nurses in almost all health related settings should feel a great deal more comfortable with the overwhelming number of females in their chosen profession. All of this research means at least that men's aversion, if any, to women colleagues at work is not solely fueled by economic considerations. This kind of aversion is of course not found in all groups of men working with women. In fact, the extent to which a man's well being is affected by the presence of a majority of women at work depends also on his family situation, as Natalie Sokoloff has shown in her study *Between Money and Love*[31].

In 2002, Evans and Steptoe conducted a study of the psychological well-being of male and female nurses. This study indicated that anxiety is associated with a high level of job strain. Such job strain became visible in the Evans and Steptoe study because sickness resulting in three to four days of absence from work was plainly related to "work hassles." The study reveals that the number of "work hassles" reported by male nurses was greater than that reported by females and that male nurses also report more sickness absences than is true of female nurses. This suggests that some of the traits heretofore believed to be of a psychological nature are in fact hormonal in nature.[32]

Status and Prestige

The National Opinion Research Center regularly publishes a scale of occupational prestige involving seventy occupations. Theses occupations are divided into "White Collar" and "Blue Collar" work. The prestige scale is based on telephone interviews with a cross section of Americans.

According to the survey published in 2001, the most prestigious jobs in America are dominated by men. Beginning with physician, the most prestigious occupation in America, the first twelve occupations range from lawyer, professor and architect to optometrist. Only then, at place 13 do we find "registered nurse" in which most employees are women. It is therefore evident that male nurses are marginal men in that they occupy an ascribed status, man as compared to woman which is higher than those with whom they work every day, while at the same time holding a job with an achieved status, nurse, which is thirteenth in the occupational prestige scale just described. This status inconsistency creates a number of tensions for men in this female dominated occupation.[33]

That status inconsistency is demonstrated by the relationship of male nurses to the male physicians they encounter daily. The tension between the two professions is of course not confined to men. Female nurses are constantly complaining that they could easily do all the procedures done by doctors and probably could do them better. We are tempted to ask whether we should close all medical schools and leave the care of the sick entirely to nurses.

Male nurses want to be considered professionals and therefore seek to establish a clear distinction between themselves and hospital aides. This is difficult because male and female nurses are often forced to perform tasks that are also part of the aides jobs. We have already seen that male nurses can seldom become part of the nurse "in-group" because of gender differences. Male nurses therefore also try to be closer to male doctors but are rejected there as well. Male doctors do not welcome male nurses into their ranks. Therefore, male nurses are excluded from all three groups working in hospitals. They are not part of the female dominated nurse work force, doctors do not want them as equals and they themselves shy away from association with male orderlies and aides.

This means that male nurses are isolates in the hospital social structure. The male nurses evidently seek over and over again to identify with doctors who don't want them and to distance themselves from nurses who resent male nurses' efforts to dissociate themselves from their profession.

Male nurses are also upset over working for a female supervisor. This of course is quite common because most nurses are women. Male nurses are also subject to allegations of homosexuality whether true or not. Female nurses are constantly complaining about the effeminate conduct of male nurses. This complaint is much more common among nurses with little formal education than those who are college graduates. The least educated female nurses assume that men become nurses because they are homosexual. Male nurses find such allegations most annoying, not because it is far less true than believed, but because allegations of homosexuality is yet another cause of their low status in the occupational scale. Nurses who come from high status families or have a college education are more likely to view nursing as undesirable for men because the pay is low and not because male nurses are homosexuals.[34]

Occupation is the most important criterion of social prestige in American society. Therefore, the position of male nurse outside the hospital setting has a great deal of influence on the self evaluation of male nurses. This indicates that most male nurses held manual or semi-skilled jobs before entering nursing which they saw as a means of attaining a professional career with more job security than they had ever had in the manual work they did previously. [35]

Subsequent to working as nurses, many of the men felt that their career aspirations could never be fulfilled because they compared themselves to doctors whose education is so far above them that they, the male nurses, cannot possibly enter the medical profession. There are of course exceptions. Yet, almost all male nurses are forced to live with the incongruity of believing they should be physicians while having far too little education to come even close to that goal.

To summarize once more the male nurse dilemma we repeat that male nurses are excluded from the female majority culture in which they work, that they shun the male aides whose work is of lesser prestige and that they cannot be doctors because they have no chance of entering that profession. Sixty percent of male nurses believe that the public does not grant nurses the prestige they deserve. This belief is true of only 20 percent of female nurses. Furthermore, only ten percent of female nurses locate themselves below the middle class but 40 percent of male nurses believe they are less than middle class.[36]

A recent survey of 310 male nurses conducted in 2002 found that 69 percent of male nurses felt that they were being stereotyped both in and out of the profession. Principally, male nurses were considered homosexuals without any evidence; further, male nurses were viewed as low achievers and lazy, leading a significant number of male nurses to the conclusion that nursing is not for men because the social consequences are so painful. These negative stereotypes extend to the male nurses families and imply that they, the male nurses, are not really men. [37]

Cognitive Dissonance

In 1957, the social psychologist Leon Festinger developed the theory of cognitive dissonance. This theory refers to the observation that something we know may be challenged by the knowledge of the opposite. Festinger goes on to show that the existence of dissonance, "being psychologically uncomfortable, will motivate the person to try to reduce the dissonance and achieve consonance." Furthermore, someone who suffers dissonance will avoid situations and knowledge which would increase his discomfort. Festinger holds that dissonance motivates people to reduce the discomfort it brings just as hungry people will seek to eat. Cognitive dissonance is therefore seen as a powerful drive like hunger, sex or thirst.[38]

Dissonance means lack of agreement. In most instances we do not face that problem. Almost everything we know is consonant with other things we also know and therefore irrelevant. For example, we know that we are a woman or a man. We engage in social work or own a business or play the piano. None of these activities conflict with our understanding of our gender role.

Male nurses, however, suffer from cognitive dissonance because they know they are men but also know that "nurse" is a word which refers to a woman and therein lies the unpleasant tension which cognitive dissonance provides.

Weinberg has listed some of the responses to cognitive dissonance experienced by homosexual men. These responses apply to male nurses as well because they are the product of dissonance and not the necessary outcome of homosexuality. The first of these is to do nothing about the dissonance tension at all. As Weinberg writes: "Some people can tolerate all kinds of ambiguities for long periods of time without particularly liking the situation in which they find themselves; nevertheless, they settle down and live with it."[39]

Denial is another means of dealing with dissonance. A male nurse can tell himself that he is really very much like a doctor and quite different from the female nurses surrounding him every day. Male nurses also deny their own feeling of status loss by joking about other male nurses and their incompetence or alleged homosexuality. As male nurses are advancing in their careers they tend to increase their efforts to deny their status and to more and more assume the pseudo doctor role. This is made easier for them as day after day patients call them "doctor" a title they do not deny even if they don't call that themselves. Theirs are lies of omission not commission.

It should be evident that men in a predominantly female occupation will be more sensitive to gender difference in communication than men working in a predominantly male environment. Therefore, men who work mostly with women will be more worried about the conversational style they use with the "opposite" gender.

Therefore it is likely that this need to worry about what one may say and how it is said will increase the tension between the sexes "on the job."[40]

The presence of male nurses creates role strain among female nurses. Socialized to play the dependent role towards male doctors, female nurses find it difficult to relate to men who perform the same functions as themselves . Here too we see how cognitive dissonance creates tensions not only for the male nurses but for the female nurses as well.

Female nurses feel consistency between their sex role and their occupational role but view the male-nurse dichotomy as inconsistent with their experience and expectations.

It is of course possible that the entrance of more and more men into nursing would eventually make the two roles so compatible that the male nurse role will eventually be viewed as normal. This has not happened yet.

In 1976, Myron Fottler studied the attitudes of female nurses towards male nurses using ten variables. That study showed conclusively that the female nurse respondents strongly disagreed with any statement indicating that male nurses might perform better than female nurses in any category. Women also rejected the idea that male nurses should receive larger salaries than women nurses because men have greater family responsibilities. Female nurses also disagreed with the assumption that men are better able to perform under pressure or that men can assume more responsibility than women. Even the belief that men are more capable of supervision was rejected by a good sized majority in the Fottler study. Female nurses also agreed that male doctors were far more willing to accept male nurses than female nurses as equals. This study reflects beliefs and attitudes nearly thirty years old today but still current among the nurses of the twenty-first century as can be ascertained by anyone who asks.[41]

Sex in the work place

Male nurses, even more than female nurses and physicians, are at risk of sexual entanglements with patients or at least with the perception that such interest may exist. For male nurses this problem has two dimensions. The first is the same as is true of all health care professionals. All need to understand how to desexualize the physical examination of patients. For homosexuals there is a second dimension. They are almost always believed to be homosexuals and some are in fact gay. Therefore male nurses must also deal with the assumption, justified or not, that their homosexual interests may be satisfied by their performance on the job. The assumption that male nurses are homosexuals is fed the public by popular entertainment. Included in such messages is ABC's *Drew Carey Show* which features a homosexual character named Oswald.

Even more pronounced in advertising homosexuality is NBC's show called *Will and Grace*. This so-called "sit-com" or situation comedy attempts to make homosexuality more acceptable than it is now. It also spreads stereotypes about homosexuals so that those truly so inclined must deal with the popular view about homosexuals as depicted in such shows.

Now as we have said, health care professionals must deal with the sexual issues of their patients. This can only be successfully achieved if the professional uses some strategies that desexualize any contact between them and the patients. Male nurses in contact with female patients are helped in desexualizing such contacts first and foremost by observing the rules and regulations or professional policies of their hospital and their professional organizations. Evidently, health care providers are prohibited from engaging in sexual relationships with patients.

In addition, male nurses and therefore all nurses and doctors are taught in school to desexualize the human body. This is done by using scientific, biomedical language for generative body parts and by approaching sex in an impersonal abstract fashion. There are also scripted methods used by doctors and nurses, both male and female, which eliminate sexual tension on examination of the nude body. One of these is to cover the body with sheets except for the area to be examined. The use of a chaperone is another and involves the presence of a female nurse as well as a male nurse if a female patient is involved. Homosexual male nurses are equally in need of a chaperone if a male patient is being examined. The reasons for the use of a chaperone vary. Some nurses say they seek to insure the comfort of the patient. This means of course that a male physician can hardly use a male nurse to examine the breasts or uterus of a female patient.[42]

Both male and female nurses who examine men seldom think of bringing a male chaperone to the examination. Men, it is believed, would be more embarrassed in the presence of a chaperone than women whose comfort is increased by the presence of a female "third party." In short, female patients are protected by chaperones and male patients are protected from chaperones. All of this is determined by arbitrary cultural beliefs which need have no application elsewhere, anymore than the belief current in Moslem countries that women must be veiled is solely the province of that culture.

In our culture, and elsewhere, it is assumed that women are more vulnerable than men and that therefore women need protection which men do not need. This assumption is patently false but can be subsumed under the oft repeated dictum that "that which people believe is real is real in its consequences." [43]

Male nurses and physicians also need a chaperone to protect them from false allegations of sexual misconduct on the part of female patients. Because such allegations need not be proved and involve the possibility of destroying a male nurse's career, such protection is vital for male nurses and physicians. Large sums of money can be recovered by making allegations of sexual assault and misconduct so that the inducement to make such charges needs to be offset by the presence of a female chaperone. Of course, homosexual patients can make accusations about male nurses and lesbian patients could make such accusations about female nurses. Such incidents are almost unknown in the profession and are therefore disregarded by female nurses. [44]

Chaperones also protect health professionals from the sexual advances by patients. Male nurses face this problem at all times because some are indeed homosexuals and all are suspected of that orientation. Evidently, this problem is particularly acute in urological examinations. Male nurses involved in such an encounter are indeed in need of protection from patient advances as are female nurses and doctors.

In addition, male nurses need to protect themselves from their own sexual feelings. Patients, both male and female can be attractive people. In our culture, men are expected to act on their sexual desires and can therefore be deemed dangerous to the health care professional. Of course female nurses and doctors can also be interested in the sexual proclivities of patients but because our culture does not allow women to act on their feelings, protection from chaperones for female nurses is deemed unnecessary.

It is assumed that male nurses could be so aroused by teenage girls that male nurses are generally discouraged from dealing with young women. Men are seen as sexual aggressors in American culture and male nurses are the victims of that belief.

Male patients often request that a male nurse catheterize them. This request is generally based on an effort to lessen the embarrassment the procedure involves. Yet, there are some men who are so homophobic that they prefer a woman nurse. In these situations female nurses are chosen as chaperones. Male nurses, in fact, are almost never chosen as chaperones for any reason.

Yet another strategy for desexualizing the patients is to objectify the patients body. The analogy used is that looking at the patients nude body is the same as looking under the hood of a car. This strategy is more easily achieved in medical school than in nursing school because medical students are taught to 'cure' while nursing students are taught to 'care.' The method employed by male nurses is to think of patients as "just another body" a method facilitated by the earlier experience in school of dissecting a cadaver.

Male nurses use the "just another body" strategy only for their female patients. The patient is then viewed as an inanimate object so that the male nurse no longer sees a sexual object but only a "thing" on which a procedure must be carried out. For many male nurses and doctors this necessary attitude leads to the accusation that they don't care about their patients because they seem so detached.

Male nurses also insure the privacy of patients, female or male, by using covers and curtains which sometimes cover all but the area to be examined. On the other hand, there are male nurses who have become so desensitized that they can examine patients in any fashion and never feel embarrassment. Nurses are taught to examine each other in training and to give each other bed baths. Such training includes learning to converse with patients about matters other than their body such as sports. Male nurses can therefore be more effective with male patients.[45]

Joking about sex is another method to desexualize the need to examine patients bodies It is used by some male nurses. This may "backfire" in that it can be interpreted as sexual harassment despite the fact that men joke about sex in "locker room" situations all the time. Such jokes serve to make any connotation of sexual interest between the male nurse and the patient ridiculous and hence of no interest. There are those who believe that a nurse who jokes about sex with patients "sets them at ease." The argument here is that joking creates "rapport" or a connection to the nurse and that jokes neutralize emotional tensions. Joking decreases the social distance between the health care worker and the patient. Most important for male nurses is the subliminal message that a man who tells sexual jokes is "straight" and not "gay" as is usually suspected.[46]

Because sexual harassment by patients is quite common, nurses and doctors may have to threaten patients who conduct themselves in that fashion. There are some patients who are already known to engage in such behavior so that nurses will approach them in a rude tone. Such rudeness serves to prevent any possibility that the patient will "get away with it." It is of course unlikely that a female patient would sexually harass a male nurse. But, because male nurses are presumed to be homosexuals, gay patients may well be inclined to do so.[47]

Summary

The sexual revolution of the 1960's led to the introduction of men into the female world of nursing. Some of the consequences of this work related status change for men have been "negative sanctions" consisting of the popular view that male nurses are not "real men" and may well be homosexuals.

These attitudes are promoted by the media but are also related to the belief that men are not suited to be in "the caring profession." Therefore, the number of men entering nursing schools has actually declined since 1995.

Male nurses are subject to occupational segregation and tokenism. Status incongruity and cognitive dissonance accompany their daily work leading to a good deal of role strain and psychological discomfort.

Notes

1.	Gerhard Falk, *Sex, Gender and Social Change: The Great Revolution,* (New York, University Press of America, 1998) p.153.

2.	Margie Johnson, Susan Goad and Britt Canada, "Attitudes towards Nursing as Expressed by Nursing and Non-nursing College Males," *Journal of Nursing Education,* 3, no.9, (November 1984):387.

3.	No author, "University of Wisconsin nursing school lures more men," *Wisconsin State Journal,* (September 13, 2004):1.

4.	Marshall Fisher, "Sex role characteristics of males in nursing." *Contemporary Nurse, 8, no.3* (1999):65-71.

5.	J. Egeland and Julie Brown, "Sex role stereotyping and role strain of male registered nurses." *Research in Nursing and Health,* 11, (1988):257-267.

6.	John Evans, "Men in nursing: issues of gender segregation and hidden advantage" *Journal of Advanced Nursing,* 26 (1997): 226-271.

7.	Philip A.. Kalisch and Beatrice Kalisch, *The Advance of American Nursing,* (Philadelphia, J.B. Lippincott Co., 1995)p.375.

8. Chris Branham, "UA addresses need for more male nurses: stereotypes abound," *Arkansas Democratic Gazette,* (July 12, 2004):1.

9. Ibid. p. 3.

10. David E. Kalist, "The gender earnings gap in the RN labor market," *Nursing Economics,* 20, no.4, (2002):155-162.

11. Christian Orlovsky, "Survey Says: Nurse Salary on the Rise," *NurseZone.Com* (November 11,2004).

12. Robert L. Anders, "Targeting Male Students," *Nurse Educator,* 18, no.2 (March/April 1993):4.

13. Roy A. Sherrod, "The Role of the Nurse-Educator when the Obstetrical Nursing Student is Male," *Journal of Nursing Education,* 28, no.8, (October 1989):377.

14. Venke Sorlie, Anders Lindseth, Reidun Forde and Astrid Norberg, "The meaning of being in ethically difficult care situations in pediatrics as narrated by male registered nurses," *Journal of Pediatric Nursing,* 18, no.5, (October 2003):350-357.

15. Susan Trossman, "Caring Knows No Gender," *The American Journal of Nursing,* 103, no. 5, (May 2003)

16. Robert K. Merton, *Social Theory and Social Structure,* New York, Free Press, (1957).

17. Charles Epstein, "Encountering the male establishment: Sex-status limits on women's careers in the professions," *American Journal of Sociology,* 75, (1970):965-992.

18. Victor Oppenheimer, "The sex labeling of jobs," *Industrial Relations,* 7, (1968):219-234.

19. Albert Muhlenkamp and John Parsons, "Characteristics of Nurses," *Journal of Vocational Behavior,* 2, (1972):261-273.

20. Bonka Boneva, "Using Email for Personal Relationships," *American Behavioral Scientists,* 45, no.3, (November 2001):530-549.

21. Rosabeth Moss Kanter, " Some Effects of Proportions on Group Life: Skewed Sex Ratios and Responses by Token Women," *American Journal of Sociology* 82, no.5. (1977):965-990.

22. John Crocker and K.M. McGraw, "What's Good for the Goose is not Good for the Gander: Social Status as an Obstacle to Occupational Achievement for Males and Females," *American Behavioral Scientist,* 27, no.3, (1984):357-369.

23. Barbara A. Gutek and B. Morasch, "Sex-Ratios, Sex-Role Spillover, and Sexual Harassment of Women at Work," *Journal of Social Issues,* 38, no.4, (1982):55-74.

24. A.G. Dworkin , J.S. Chafetz and R. Dworkin, "The Effects of Tokenism on Work Alienation," *Work and Occupation,* (August 1986).

25.   Heidi Hartman, "Capitalism, Patriarchy and Job Segregation by Sex, in: M. Blaxall and B.B. Reagan, Editors. *Women and the Workplace,* (Chicago, University of Chicago Press, 1976)pp.137-69.

26.   Michael D. Orlansky and William L. Heward, *Voices: Interviews with Handicapped People,* (Columbus, Merrill, 1981)pp.133-134.

27.   Kenneth Plummer, "Misunderstanding Labeling Perspectives," in David Downes and Paul Rock, Editors, *Deviant Interpretations,* (London:Martin Robertson, 1979)p. 85-121.

28.   Talcott Parsons, "Age and Sex in the Social Structure of the United States," in Logan Wilson and William L. Kolb, Editors, *Sociological Analysis,* (New York: Harcourt, Brace and Co. 1949):598.

29.   Lilianne Floge and Deborah M. Merrill, "Tokenism Reconsidered: Male Nurses and Female Physicians in a Hospital Setting," *Social Forces,* 64, (1986): 925-947.

30.   Scott J .South, Charles M. Bonjean, William T. Markham and Judy Corder, "Social Structure and Inter-group Interaction: Men and Women of the Federal Bureaucracy," *American Sociological Review,* 47(1982): 587-589.

31.   Natalie Sikoloff, *Between Money and Love,* (New York, Praeger, 1990).

32.   Olga Evans and Andrew Steptoe, "The contribution of gender role orientation, work factors and home stressors to psychological well-being and sickness absence in male and female dominated occupational groups," *Social Science and Medicine,* 54, no. 4(*Social Science and Medicine,* February 4, 2002):481-492.

33.   John J. Macionis, *Society: The Basics,* (Upper Saddle River, N.J., Prentice Hall, 2004)p.203.

34.   Robert Merton, *Social Theory and Social Structure,* (Glencoe, Ill. The Free Press, 1957)p. 305.

35.   Herbert Hyman, "The Value Systems of Different Classes," in: Reinhard Bendix and Seymour Martin Lipset, Editors, *Class, Status and Power,* (New York; The Free Press, 1966)p.488.

36.   Bernard E. Segal, "Male Nurses: A Case Study in Status Contradiction and Prestige Loss," *Social Forces,* 41, no. 1 (October 1962):31-38.

37.   Murray Fisher, "Stereotypes of male nurses live on," *Nursing Review, no.3* (March 2002):

38.   Leon Festinger, *A Theory of Cognitive Dissonance,* (Stanford, Cal. Stanford University Press, 1957)p. 3.

39.   Thomas S. Weinberg, *Gay Men, Gay Selves,* (New York: Irvington Publishers, 1983)p.101

40.   Christine L. Williams and e. Joel Heikes, *Gender and Society,* 7, no.2 (June 1993):284.

41.   Myron D. Fottler, "Attitudes of Female Nurses Toward the Male Nurse: A Study of Occupational Segregation," *Journal of Health and Social Behavior,* 17, no. 2, (June 1976):98-110.

42.   Patti A. Giuffre and Christine L. Williams, "Not Just Bodies: Strategies for Desexualizing the Physical Examination of Patients," *Gender and Society,* 14, no.3, (June 2000): 457-482.

43.   John J. Macionis, *Society: The Basics,* (Upper Saddle River, N.J., 2004)p.90.

44.   Ibid. p.464.

45.   Ibid. 472.

46.   Karyn Buxman,"Make room for laughter," *American Journal of Nursing,* 91, (December 1991):46-51.

47.   Victor Schultz, "Reconceptualizing sexual harassment," *Yale Law Journal,* 107, (1998):1683-1805

Chapter VII
Summary and Conclusion

It is common knowledge that every occupation/profession has members who deviate from the norm and standards of their chosen field. Nurses are not the exception. The difference is that the nursing profession is one of those that deal with the lives of human beings. Improper care can result in tragedy, pain and death. The reactions of these professionals, both positive and negative, make a serious difference for those for whom they are responsible. Their outlook and behavior is essential in carrying out their tasks as they minister to the ill and the helpless.

We are not including here the majority of well meaning caring individuals who have chosen their profession because they feel deeply for people, are eager to help and chose this very necessary and important role with sincerity and a love for humanity "one person at a time." Most nurses fall into the above category and are responsible and respectable folk. Here too are not included those nurses who have made an occasional accidental error since there is no one alive who does not make mistakes. It should also be remembered that those in less vulnerable positions can make mistakes which will do no lasting harm to anyone.

We must closely examine the motivations, the thoughts, ideas and actions of those who have fallen into the category of deviant nurses. They are individuals of varying ages from very young to old; from those with the minimum educational requirements for their chosen field to those with advanced degrees; for those who are of superior intelligence and those who are of average or a little more than average intellect; for those who have religious affiliation and those who do not; for individuals with strong convictions and others who have few or none. We have in these chapters attempted to study and isolate the characteristics of nurses who have failed to demonstrate the expectations generally anticipated of those who have chosen to become and are employed in the profession of nursing.

When we look at the nurses who have engaged in serious deviant behavior, we find that a number of them have come from dysfunctional families where drug and alcohol dependency was a part of their lifestyle; where abusive behavior including neglect and sometimes abandonment was directed and included in the lives of their children. These children now adults entered the profession frequently for the wrong reasons and rationalizations as have been seen in the examples cited. A number of these individuals are known to have "anti-social" personalities. They consistently and often place their own deprivations, unmet needs and interests above those of others and use their patients as their targets. These folks act and react in ways that have been learned at their proverbial mother's knee or the absence of this knee.

All names that will be mentioned in this chapter are fictitious ones but (as they are in all of the pages of this book) the characteristics and descriptions are real and have been studied, researched and observed over a period of fifteen years. The cases cited in this chapter have been categorized according to backgrounds, personalities, attitudes, situations, behaviors and problem areas that have reoccurred in people who have been viewed as deviant from the norms and expectations of the skilled and caring professionals that are known as nurses! The cases summarized below are individuals who have exhibited the major forms and types of deviant behavior that have been described and exhibited throughout this book. These are all individuals with human frailties and behaviors which are not acceptable in society and definitely not in the caring professionals that we know as nurses.

Jane is a young woman who always wanted to emulate her mother including her mother's profession. She was told from a young child until she graduated from high school that she would become a nurse. Although she knew in some vague fashion what was expected of her she could not quite understand the entire situation. Her grades were not much more than C's and the studies were difficult for her. She struggled very hard to get by in nursing school. She barely made it through the Practical Nurse Program. When she got a position in a nursing home as a nurses aide since she had not yet passed the licensure examination. She attempted to take the test several times. After failing for a third time she left her home town having learned through a former classmate that a place existed in Redwood Township that would issue a license without having to pass an examination and that would only require a fee of one thousand dollars to give out such a license and with which she could practice as a licensed practical nurse. The document that she received from this "school" looked authentic and appeared flawless with Jane's name, State and other alleged verifications printed in amazingly creative lettering. She framed this piece of paper almost instantly and obtained a job in a small town hospital, a considerable distance from the city of her birth. In the beginning of her work the woman who had hired her and the other staff were thrilled to have such a pleasant and attractive colleague in their midst. She was very accommodating and agreeable and was willing to work any shift assigned. She extended herself to the Aides, taught them how to make a comfortable bed and made a number of friends among them. There was a big problem. She was confused about the drugs needed for specific patients and was often confused. It did not take long before she made her first drug error. She was not even aware that she had made this. When it was discovered she was defensive and somewhat apologetic at the same time. She also did not know the various techniques that were necessary such as giving insulin injections properly in a timely fashion; ascertaining that the correct dosages of drugs be dispensed and for what reason. She was afraid to ask questions because she was guilty about her lack of knowledge since she had claimed she possessed more experience than was actually true. She could not even ask her mother questions since she had not shared with her that she had obtained a "license" fraudulently. Many of her errors were the result of her fears and anxieties. After six month on the job she got a number of warnings and was ultimately dismissed from her position. Here we see a young woman who was unable to achieve her objectives in the time that she wanted. She was not a good candidate for her profession because of her poor learning record and additionally she had chosen a field to please her mother, not altogether for a healthy reason. In her situation she was unable to grasp what needed to be done to become a qualified nurse. She brought much discomfort and pain to her unsuspecting patients and supported a fraudulent operation in addition to her own dishonest behavior.

Daryl always had big dreams. His goal was to be a success. He felt strongly that the most prestigious position of all would be was to become a physician. From the time he was a young boy he loved his pediatrician and all that he stood for. Daryl's parents encouraged him and bought him a small stethoscope set with which he played doctor and he would examine his brother and sister and later some of the children with whom he played. It was fun for him and gave him the feeling of power and superiority. He was in charge and he felt good about himself. He held that dream of doctoring throughout his high school years. When he entered college he took some science courses along with the liberal arts requirements which were a part of his curriculum. He had some excellent grades in English and History but Chemistry was very difficult for him. Mathematics also presented some difficulties for him and he achieved a "gentleman's" C in that subject. Upon graduation from college he did manage to have a cumulative average of "B." He applied to a number of medical schools but was not accepted. Every time he received a rejection letter he became progressively more discouraged. It did not take too long before he decided to enter a School of Nursing. He was one of two males who were in his classes and although he felt somewhat uncomfortable with the thirty five females in the group he comforted himself with the knowledge that he would have contact with his idols the physicians. He was helpful to the women in his class, assisted them when strength was an asset during his clinical training and he did become friendly with the other male students. The discomfort that he felt in the beginning was ameliorated by his feelings of superiority and specialness and his ability to add an extra dimension to the profession. He was successful in graduating and did well in the licensing examination. He managed to get a position in a large hospital and always wore a white coat. He enjoyed being called "Doc" and he was frequently mistaken for a physician which he greatly enjoyed. He made it a point not to correct the patients when they called him by that name and he told his friends that he knew more than most doctors. He spoke frequently about his unique skills, about his patients and their maladies, and what he did to ameliorate their pain and how he cured their illnesses. On several occasions he did not follow the M.D's orders and changed the course of the treatments. It was during several of these ministerings of drugs that a patient became very ill and unresponsive. He had changed one medication for another and had administered a strong dosage to the patient. The man was close to death and somehow it was discovered that "Doc" had taken matters into his own hands. Fortunately the patient survived but much damage had been done. "Doc" had been closely observed for some time prior to the occurrence in question and after the last very serious episode he was deleted from the staff with other consequences that followed.

Mary was a very ambitious young woman who worked diligently to get excellent marks in high school. She had come from a middle class family who had high ambitions for their children. They wanted them all to have upward mobility, to become wealthy and not to have to struggle to earn a livelihood like they had done. The two boys were encouraged to succeed in their studies and the girl was encouraged to find a "rich" man who would adulate her and keep her in a style to which she was not accustomed. It was Mary's mother who encouraged her daughter to strive to better herself and suggested that her daughter find a career that would bring her together with men of accomplishment or men who had potential. Mary agreed wholeheartedly and decided that she would become a nurse, meet physicians and marry one of them. While attending nursing school she was a bit disappointed since there was little opportunity to get close to physicians especially while she was training in a nursing facility where she only once fleetingly saw an elderly male physician who was dictating his findings on a medical chart. Although she was a capable person her energies were more engaged in concentrating on finding a suitable marriage partner than in her essential performance. She did work hard because she knew that was the only possible way of achieving her long term goal. After graduating from nursing school she managed to obtain a job in a hospital and where her opportunity for meeting physicians was good. She was kind to the patients and did the tasks assigned her but was easily distracted when medical students, interns and other young physicians were in her vicinity. She was disappointed when she learned that the majority of these gentlemen were married or engaged but she continued to have hopes that she would find one that was not so involved. After a long concerted effort Mary (teased by the other young nurses and nicknamed Marry) managed to attract Peter, a thirty year old doctor who paid attention to her. He flirted with her, invited her for a drink and she enjoyed his company. What did happen with this young woman was that she began to become less interested in her patients and her duties and concentrated on her relationship with Dr. Peter. She was very much enamored with him. She would daydream about her happy life with him, the children they would produce and the wealth and luxury that she would have. In her thoughts she would decorate a multi million dollar home, would be envied by all other women and would have a life like a movie princess, only better. Thus preoccupied Mary made many medication errors. She was careless and paid little attention to the tasks and duties at hand. At first her errors were not noticed, then several were overlooked and two were even attributed to another nurse who had worked with Mary. It was on one of the shifts that a medication error was made that did not go unnoticed. Thus Mary was "written up" and very closely observed following this incident. Many more medication errors occurred and ultimately Mary lost her opportunity to succeed in the her chosen field. (Incidentally it was later learned that Peter did not marry her since he was already involved with another woman.) It is obvious in this case that Mary entered the field of nursing for reasons other than having passion or sincere interest in her profession.

Adeline a very attractive forty two year old woman whose career, husband three children and house work kept her very busy. Already as a child she was an over achiever. "Addie," as she was nicknamed, was the oldest of six siblings and she was expected to assist and take over the care of the younger ones when her mother was too busy. Her father a factory worker spent many of his weekends in a bar, drinking with his friends thus placing much of the home responsibilities on his wife. She in turn confided in her oldest daughter and counted on her for help. When Addie grew up she managed to get a partial scholarship to a nursing school and was thrilled when the capping ceremony took place and when she ultimately received her registered nursing status. Adeline worked very hard and "juggled" her duties skillfully. Her spouse, a salesman, was frequently out of town, therefore she took a job on the night shift. This enabled her to be available for her offspring during the day and tend to the multitudinous chores which were always awaiting her attention. Leisure time was non existent for her and the few hours of sleep that were available to her were frequently interrupted by phone calls and other demands.

After a time Adeline was promoted to night supervisor in the nursing facility where she was an employee. There were many nights when she felt exhausted and as she described it "bone tired." Her husband also became critical of her and felt neglected. Because their children were left unsupervised when Thomas, her husband, was out of town, her teen aged son began to exhibit some delinquent behavior in school. He had too many absences, feigned illness, and he was said to have little respect for one of his female teachers. An additional burden was now placed upon Adeline as she had to intervene at her son's school and she spent much time getting outside help for him and spending time which was something of which she had so little. Her husband was not there to help her and all the problems seemed to Addie to rest on her "shoulders." Thomas seemed to spend too many nights on the road and Adeline suspected that he was unfaithful. All of these situations were overwhelming to the nurse. She felt that she needed something to relax and to quell her anxiety. Since she had access to the medication cabinet she helped herself to a narcotic which was left from a patient who was no longer in the institution. Having ingested that she felt some relief from the overwhelming pressures which were so much a part of her life. As time went on Addie's habit grew and her problems seemed not so difficult to bear. With her addiction other difficulties began. At times she felt very tired during her midnight shift, she felt unable to stay awake and she would nod in her office. At other times she would become very energetic and demanding of the staff and expect great things from them. She was also known to place some of her responsibilities on the other workers on that shift. If they did not meet her demands she would become angry and vituperative toward them. She would make them feel inadequate which would cause anger and they would exhibit uncooperative behavior. Her mood would fluctuate from night to night. Even during the day she was not functioning with her usual energy and at times she seemed inebriated. When her husband was at home she became openly accusatory which created much strife in the home. Addie's life became more chaotic than ever. The stress that she had attempted to alleviate had escalated. Because the staff found working with Adeline difficult several of her supervisors reported her to the Director of Nursing. This woman in turn observed Addie very closely and one evening she was found diverting drugs. This very hard working, conscientious woman was harmed by circumstances which seemed to be beyond her control. It was fortunate both for Adeline and for those around her that she was terminated from her employment before too much damage was done. Although her nursing license was suspended she became involved in rehabilitation and ultimately she found much solace and help for herself and for her children.

Chester and Harold were two male nurses who had been friends since early childhood. Chester enjoyed the sciences and wanted to have an occupation that involved his interests and that would make his working life an enjoyable one. He did not want to be "one of the common herd" who went to a job every day that he hated. Thus he decided to become a lab technician since he only needed very little training to engage in this endeavor. It was only a short time before "Chet" found his position too routine. He wanted something that would challenge him more. Seeing that his friend Harold was enrolled in a School of Nursing and was near completion of his studies he questioned him about his learnings, the clinical aspects of the schooling.

Harold was very enthusiastic and "upbeat" about his soon to be occupation. He had no aversion about being a minority in his class and enjoyed his contact with the eager young women with whom he could exchange information and experiences about the hospital in which they had their practical training. After much discussion with Harold and seeing his attitude toward his studies Chester decided to apply to Nursing School. Academically he had no problems with the curriculum but he did have some qualms when it came to the clinical part of his practice. He did get accustomed to what had to be done and eventually enjoyed his contact with both teachers, hospital staff and patients. He was not squeamish about the human body and body fluids, the witnessing of the serious damage to the folks who were brought in by ambulance to the emergency room. He was well accepted by his classmates and cohorts. He graduated with honors and proudly received his license after taking the examination once. Chester was employed in the same hospital for two years when some problems arose that were being investigated by this nurse's supervisor. On his floor on the evening shift a young male patient complained that he had been "groped" in the genital area by a person who was examining him. His illness and surgery had no bearing upon his penis and he was unsure whether the examiner was a physician or a nurse. The room was fairly dark since it was night and the patient was tired and had been sedated for pain prior to this episode. All staff who had been on the shift that evening were questioned and there was a denial by all who had been working that night. When Chester was asked what he knew about the situation he adamantly denied any problem. He stated that he had come into the room to tend to any needs that the patient might have but he did not examine him other than taking his vital signs. The allegation was dismissed but it was six months later when a similar event occurred on the shift which included Chester. This time the family of a young patient in question was involved and the actions pointed toward Chester. He was seen by one of the aide's spending much time in the young male patient's room and the aide heard the boy cry out for help. Despite the fact that Chester adamantly denied any wrong doing and any problem with any of the patients his denials were no longer credible.

After a session with the supervisor, the Director of Nursing and the Hospital Administrator it was decided to terminate Chester's employment from the staff. After reporting the incident to the State's Board of Nursing his license to practice nursing was ultimately revoked.

Monita Kram was born into a very dysfunctional household. Her mother was a single young woman who knew nothing about child care nor did she have an interest in this pursuit. She viewed the little girl as one would a toy but her interest ceased when the baby cried. The Mom lived on welfare and "needed a man to help her out." She found a number of men that she met in bars who enjoyed her company for a night or two and one even did come home with her. Monita was frequently left with neighbors and even left alone in the small disheveled apartment that was rented to welfare recipients. The "gentleman" that did come to stay with the child's Mom disliked children and had no use for "Nita" as her mother called her. Alcohol seemed to be more important than food in the Kram household thus the child was not nourished well and at times being hungry she had long periods of crying as a young baby. She seemed to have been suffering from cholic. The screaming, as Ms. Kram labeled the wails, disturbed the woman's boyfriend even more than it did the Mom. At those times they would roll Nita's second hand bassinet into the bathroom and engage in their alcoholic and sexual activities. Thus little Nita was uncared for and neglected. As the child grew she was frequently left to her own devices. At age six the little girl was placed in a foster home where a number of other children were housed. Nita missed her mother and frequently daydreamed of being held, cuddled and loved. This did not happen. When Nita started school she had some difficulties in the beginning but she was very eager to learn and her teacher, a very kind and sympathetic woman was very fond of the little girl and her eagerness to learn. This was a real impetus and change for the child and she looked forward to leaving the foster home every morning to receive the approval and frequent accolades of Mrs. Jones, her teacher. The child's mother rarely came to see her and when she did appear she often brought the boyfriend and paid more attention to him even during the brief times that she spent with Nita. She would bring her an occasional little trinket which the child would touch and cherish when the mother was gone. She would cuddle the toy, would speak to it and cradle it the way that she would like to have been cradled. She missed the nurturing that she so yearned for and she would frequently retreat into her own thoughts, into her own world where love was plentiful and she was cared about. She had several bouts of illness during school when she was sent to the school nurse. This woman treated the child very well and she would frequently stop into the small office of Nurse Chubbs and speak a few words to her. Monita admired the nurse so much and at age eight she already knew what she wanted to be. Nurse Chubbs was such a warm, caring person who seemed to make "everything all right." She was able to take away the worries and pains that the little girl had, at least for a while. As Nita grew older she excelled in school, her grades were always good and she enjoyed the positive comments and feelings that these accomplishments brought. She was well liked by most of her teachers and she graduated from high school with honors. It was not long before she enrolled in a School of Nursing. She felt good during her clinical practice when she could take care of the patients and they in turn responded very well to this eager young woman who was so kind and showed so much warmth and caring. Again, just as she had done in grade and high school she graduated with honors. Monita succeeded to get a job in a large hospital. The patients under her care were happy with their nurse and always got a smile when she entered their room. As time passed a new wing was opened adjacent to the hospital where long term care for brain injured patients was established. It was a more lucrative position with a considerable higher wage than Nita was receiving. She applied and managed to be hired for the position. In the beginning Nita enjoyed the fact that she had been chosen over a number of other applicants but her feeling of exuberance was short lived. She lost her excitement since she felt the patients gave back very little. Their responses were sparse often bizarre and frightening to her. One young man who had been in a motorcycle accident let out some curdling screams. Somehow this man reminded her of her mother's latest lover – he seemed to look like him. A woman who had a major and severe spinal cord injury was very demanding in her own way. There was no one in that unit where Nita worked that seemed to return her smile, a smile which was very rare since she had begun this job. She seemed to get no response from the people that she serviced. There was no hug, no kind word just very ill, in her mind very frightening and ungiving people. She seemed to be reliving her own deprived childhood where there was no mothering, nothing for her, no comfort, only rejection and loneliness. In addition she had a supervisor who was very aloof and demanding of her supervisees and to Nita it felt that she was isolated for abuse from this nurse. Monita began to become inefficient and neglectful toward her charges. She at times "forgot" to inject insulin into the woman that had the severe stroke, at other times she injected too much. She also seemed to be "somewhere else" staring absent mindedly into space, not responding to her current environment. She looked pained. She felt helpless and seemed to be unable to extricate herself from her present situation. She dreaded going to work every day and took time off to curl up in her bedroom with an "unexplainable illness." This went on for a time until she was called before the Director of Nursing since she had neglected her patients, had not treated the decubitus of one man, not medicated several others properly nor in a timely fashion and had not adhered to the infection control directives. The severe reprimand that she felt increased her feelings of being disliked and eventually she was terminated from her position. Monita was a woman who became a nurse because mothering and nursing were closely related in her mind. She wanted and needed the love that her mother never gave her. In nursing/mothering the patients, she lived vicariously. She was not only the nurse-mother but also was being mothered by the patients who loved and responded to her. When she placed herself in a position that did not afford her the affection and caring that she needed she regressed to the rejected motherless little girl that could not function as an adult nor as the giving, caring mother nurse that she wanted so sincerely to be.

Kashiva was enrolled in a Practical Nursing Program during her last two years in high school. Her guidance counselor had given her a vocational aptitude test and she had scored above average for Nursing. After graduation she studied hard to take her licensure examination. She failed the first time since her language skills were not the best and some of the questions were not understood by her. She did succeed on the second try. Kashiva called "Kash" by her friends had been raised in an impoverished household with two parents who had difficulty supporting their seven children. Kash was the oldest of the group and she was eager to get a job and to be able to afford the material things of which she had been deprived. Nursing seemed to offer her that opportunity. Her first position was at a nursing home where she was assigned to a wing of elderly people who were in various stages of the aging process, of frailties both physically and cognitively. There were among them men and women who were incapable of recalling their own identity. Some had families who would visit them and others no longer had relatives or were abandoned and alone except for the staff of the institution in which they found themselves. Kash followed instructions as given her by her supervisor and made her charges as comfortable as possible. She had a routine which she followed which she had learned during her time in school. She was very proud of her name plate with her LPN insignia which she attached to the front of her uniform. She liked it when she was addressed as "Nurse" by the patients who called her by that title. She could barely believe that she had achieved her goal and that she had some money in her wallet with which could buy some of the things that she needed and wanted. As time went by her desires became greater and she realized that her checks were not as high as she at first believed. She wanted certain items that she could not afford on the earnings that were hers. She frequently compared herself to others in the nursing home – people who spoke of lobster dinners delicacies and other scarce and expensive food items that she had never tasted or experienced. She heard other young nurses speak about their well off families, their generous boyfriends and material things that she could never afford. Kash became envious of others who seemed to have so much more than she had ever had. She pondered about how she could better her earning power, increase her acquisitions and lead a more comfortable life. She felt the internal pressure to have as much or more as she believed her peers had as well as the families of patients who were well dressed and allegedly affluent. One day when a family came in with a package of new underwear as well as several colorful blouses which she admired she decided she would help herself to one of each since they would not be missed by the recipient, an elderly cognitively impaired woman. She did succeed in this endeavor and no one seemed to notice that these items were missing. Kashiva was very skilled in hiding her "loot" hiding them under some towels and later transferring them to her large lunch container that she owned and kept in the staff's locker room in her personal locker. There were a number of other opportunities that this nurse used to her advantage. Despite signs that valuables and moneys should be kept in the facilities front office for safe keeping there were some residents who did not adhere to this directive and kept their money in their room. Mrs. Griffin was one of those, a woman cared for by Kashiva. One night shift when the patient was sleeping the nurse quietly opened the drawer in which Mrs. Griffin had stashed five twenty dollar bills and two one dollar ones. Kashiva helped herself to twenty dollars which she stuffed into her brassier. She felt certain that no one would notice that anything was awry. The next day when the patient counted her treasure she was certain that something was missing. She was sure that she had one hundred and two dollars which now turned to eighty two. She questioned herself, could she possibly have miscalculated or had she not? She plagued herself for a long time before she reported this to the day nurse. This innocent young nurse felt accused but reported Mrs. Griffin's allegation to her supervisor. The latter pondered the situation for a time and then decided that no doubt the patient was mistaken and possibly confused and nothing further was said. (This is not an infrequent stance that is taken by the nursing home staff since they are convinced that the patient is confused, senile or merely forgetful. Therefore accusations are often negated and not considered as seriously as they should be.) Kash felt secure and safe that she would not be suspected and no one would discover the thefts that occurred at her hands. As time went on Kashiva felt safe and felt good that she had money to spend that was really "hers" since "the old lady didn't need it anyway" and additionally she serviced this woman who she considered wealthy and who could not enjoy her possessions in any event. Now that she had succeeded she felt more courageous. She had no pangs of conscience since she believed herself disadvantaged while others had more than they needed and to Kashiva these other people seemed to have lived in splendor. It was noticed by various lucid patients and family members that at times new or near new items of clothing were missing from one resident or another. Sometimes these losses were reported at other times they were not. Everyone seemed to be suspect. When Kashiva was questioned along with other staff members she stated that many of these patients are senile and can't recall what they owned and at other times she alleged that possibly the laundry had either lost the items in question or that other residents had entered the patients rooms and had carried the items to their rooms or to other patients rooms. This was easily believable because there were instances that these actions occurred. Since to date there had been no dire consequences for the thefts that the nurse perpetrated she became very brave. One night she entered the room of one of her patients during the midnight shift. There was only a night light in this double room and both of the inhabitants were asleep. Kashiva's nursing shoes cushioned the sounds that are ordinarily made when individuals ambulate. She had noticed some time ago that Risa, the resident in question owned a beautiful diamond and emerald ring that her late husband had given her when they were engaged. Risa felt comforted and close to her beloved spouse and would frequently touch it with her other hand like one does a shaman, a rabbit foot or a good luck charm. The ring had been admired by all and to Kash it was something that she wanted very much. She thought about the glittering stone with its deep green shimmering emeralds and felt that some day she could either wear it or sell it and she would feel "rich" and would be envied by all who knew her. The temptation was great to "dispossess" this resident of her treasure. As Kashiva felt the ring on Risa's hand that night she attempted to get it off the resident's finger. It was very difficult to turn since it was very tight on Risa's hand and it took a great deal of effort to move and twist that ring even a small fraction of an inch. The pain that was created by the force used to extricate the jewelry caused Risa to moan. She seemed to be in pain and had an awareness that something was happening to her. Since she was in somewhat of a hynogogic state she was not totally consciously aware of the reality around her. Kash stealthily walked out of the room angry at herself for not having been able to extricate that fabulously "rich" ring from the resident's hand. She was determined to succeed on her next try. It was only a few nights later when Kashiva made another effort to repeat the performance. Only this time she took with her a jar of Vaseline. She worked this into the finger of the patient and with many revolutions of the band she ultimately was able to remove the ring from Risa's hand. She placed the treasure into the pocket of her uniform and covered it with a tissue. The next day Risa felt her left hand and noticed that her ring was missing. Her finger was swollen and pained. She cried out and one of the day nurses came into the room and questioned the weeping Risa about her problem. When the nurse looked at the woman's hand she saw that the finger was swollen and that the ring was missing. The first thing she did was search the room. She searched the adjacent bathroom, the window sills, the shower stand, the water closet and the medicine cabinet. She questioned Risa and wondered whether the resident had misplaced the ring, whether it might have fallen into the toilet bowl, whether it was in one of her drawers, possibly under some clothing, etc. Many questions were asked and when Risa's son came to visit he reported the theft to the nursing supervisor. Everyone was questioned and no one recalled anything of any consequence except an aide. She had observed nurse Kashiva entering the resident's room and did not see her come out again. This indicated to the aide that it took a long time to do whatever was being accomplished. She also heard the moans of Risa coming from her room. She was uncertain whether the noise came from the roommate or from Risa. After many questionings and denials on the part of the staff including Kashiva, a police detective was called. After speaking with the administrator he advised that Kashiva should be closely monitored and followed. She was promptly removed to another wing of the nursing facility. For several months nothing remarkable was seen on the shift where Kashiva worked. A half year passed when this nurse was seen taking a package of new, unmarked underwear from a patient's drawer and stuffing it into the front of the slacks of her nursing uniform. She was almost instantly confronted by the nursing supervisor who asked her to leave the premises at once under surveillance. Kashiva's nursing career thus ended!

In reviewing and summarizing each chapter in this book we find the following: The Introduction described the Nature of Deviance, the various theories of that term, and the major proponents of these theories are here explained in sociological terms. It includes the labeling theory which alleges that nothing is considered deviant unless it is labeled as such. Other scholars defined deviance as "conduct which is thought to require the attention of social control agencies." An act of deviance is also defined as an act which is contrary to the norm. (There are cultures and groups of people whose norms differ from those of the norms as seen by the middle class of America.). Because the large majority of nurses are caring and trusted people that are thought of highly by the public, the unacceptable behavior that is seen is out of the norm of expectations. The nurses thus described in this chapter illustrate the concept of deviance among those who have chosen the profession of nursing.

Chapter II gives a detailed analysis of the profession of nursing: The numerical size of that profession and what it entails to be a nurse, to practice, the standards, the tasks, the expectations. It describes the limitless duties that must be performed, the skills that are needed, the meticulousness that is essential. Nurses must be leaders and followers. They must adhere to the physicians orders but must use their intellectual abilities to carry out tasks and duties that are not prescribed when the situation calls for such judgment. They must teach the nurses aides and families when and where indicated and must have the ability to do so. They must be able to get along with people, remain calm under crisis conditions, to be attentive to their charges and work hard and fast, often giving to others before they think of themselves. They must dispense medication accurately and in a timely fashion. In this chapter also an analysis is made of nurses backgrounds, their personalities, their goals, their objectives; what their needs are, their desires, their abilities; how they are trained and educated – their curriculum. Here their opportunities for employment are examined, how they view themselves, their colleagues, their peers, their patients and their responsibilities. How they are similar or different from each other, their uniqueness. How they differ from those in other professions and careers. All of these factors are viewed in order to enable us to know and understand what nursing in the twenty-first century entails and why and how the unexpected happens. Here too are described the different levels of nursing from the licensed practical to the registered nurse, their level of training and their similar and differing tasks and responsibilities. It describes the examinations that they have taken to reach their goal and the educational requirements that are needed. Here too the salaries are viewed and what nurses can expect to earn at the various stages of their careers and the positions that they hold within these careers. Included here are the steps that can be attained within each level of responsibility from "floor" nurse, to supervisor, to nurse manager, to Director of nursing to Administrator. Also here can be included the nurses who are employed by drug companies who utilizes nurses to sell their products. The changing roles of the nurse via the physician during this century are delineated and examined. Nurse practitioners have become a noticeable part of the American scene. They are called on and are able to act in lieu of the traditional healer and are able to write prescriptions which was formerly a task only a licensed Medical Doctor was permitted to perform. Reimbursement and insurance situations are here discussed as are other important aspects of the changing scene inside the medical profession of which nurses are an integral part.

Chapter III "The Perpetrators" describes the nurses who have committed unacceptable acts which have in some way been injurious to patients. Although the names of these nurses have been withheld as have the names of the places where these deviances took place, the nurses are real people and actual cases described and analyzed in the case studies presented. They are individuals who worked in hospitals and nursing homes. Their characters are examined and complete histories and examinations of their uniqueness and their differences are here cited. They are folks who appeared before a three to five member jury, all members of a State Board of Nursing. They sometimes were accompanied by their private attorney, sometimes not. Present was also a prosecutor, as well as a second attorney appointed by the State, as well as a court stenographer who recorded all conversations within the hearings in question.

Chapter IV discusses the flawed moral character of nurses who have because of their lack of conscience been apprehended because of unethical, dishonest and indecent practices. These included practitioners who used street and non prescribed narcotic drugs; those who indulged in theft as well as those who were alcoholics. Their flaws involved their functioning as nurses and impacted on their actions and behaviors in their job performance and their ability to carry out the very important functions to which they were assigned.

"The More Vulnerable Ones" are the nurses described in Chapter V. Discussed here are the numbers of people in this country who died due to preventable in-hospital errors. The cost involved in these errors are enormous to say nothing of the cost to the individuals who lost their lives due to these mistakes. These problems are created by physicians, pharmacists, other health care professionals as well as nurses. Here discussed are the errors made by nurses and the lack of caring shown by the individuals involved. Among others, errant prison nurses are described in detail and their actions which because of their attitudes and behaviors caused the death of prisoners under their care. Here is pointed out the need of supervision, the need of compassion, the serious effects that negative and judgmental attitudes can have and how these attitudes are played out in behaviors. It points out how important the need for positive, professional relationships between prison guards and nurses are -which is an essential aspect for the ongoing well being of the prisoners. Knowledge of applied psychology is very helpful for preventing the suffering and potential harm for both prisoners and staff. The prison nurse must make some knowledgeable and difficult decisions in the confines of the prison since medical doctors are rarely physically available at a moments notice. In this chapter is also described the vulnerability of the elderly in hospitals and nursing facilities. Because of their frailties and multiple needs and infirmities both physically and cognitively, the elderly are not too often given the care that all humans deserve regardless of their age and stage of life classification. Negligence of care in nursing homes has been known to include over or under medicating, also known for falls and for bed sores. The cases in this section of the book were patients who because of their vulnerability were physically and/or morally wounded.

Chapter VI describes male nurses, the struggles they are facing, their attitudes, positions and problems in the female world in which they find themselves. It gives the history of their beginnings in the field of nursing. It describes their motivation, their ambitions, their needs. It differentiates the uniqueness between themselves and their female counterparts. There is still a certain aura of stigma attached to the male in an erstwhile female profession. Also discussed is the salary differential between male and female nurses. Men who have entered the nursing profession frequently suffer from criticism and suspicion. They have been known to have an inclusion problem, meaning they are excluded from the group to which they belong since a number of female nurses have shown decidedly negative attitudes toward them and have rejected them as equals among their professional compatriots. Examined in this segment of the book are the kinds of deviances that have been exhibited by the male nurses which have been seen by supervisors, directors of nursing, administrators in hospitals and other health care facilities.

It is the fervent hope of these authors that a great deal can be achieved to prevent a large number of the problems that have been encountered in the field of nursing. This can be done through education, careful screenings of potential candidates for admission to schools of nursing; through a closer examination of motives and ambitions, through careful history taking of student applicants and a closer examination of the licenses and the unqualified "schools" that give out fraudulent licenses. Before being admitted to be qualified, candidates should be closely supervised to determine whether they have the expertise to perform the tasks and duties that their very important job demands!

Bibliography

Aiken, Lorraine, "Transformation of the nursing workforce," *Nursing Outlook*, Vol.43, No.5, 1995.

American Association of Colleges of Nursing, "Baccalaureate nursing education for the future: Defining the essential elements," Washington, D.C., 1997.

Anders, Robert L., "Targeting Male Students," *Nurse Educator*, 18, no.2 (March/April 1993).

Anders, Robert L., "Targeting Male Students," *Nurse Educator*, Vol. 18, No.2, March/April, 1993.

Anderson, Carole A., "Nurses to Recommend Provider Mix in Shortage Areas," *Public Health Reports*, Vol. 113, No. 1, January/February 1998.

Anderson, Ruth R. and Reuben A. McDaniel, Jr., "Intensity of Registered Nurse Participation in Nursing Home Decision Making," *The Gerontologist*, Vol.38, No.1, February 1998.

Andriote, John Manuel, "The 1998 Survey," *Working Woman*, February 1998.

Associated Press, "Syracuse nursing students seek lawyer in administrative mix-up," *The Buffalo News*, August 11, 1998.

Beck, Cheryl Tatano, "Nursing Students' Experiences Caring for Dying Patients," *Journal of Nursing Education*, Vol. 36, No.9, November 1997.

Boneva, Bonka, "Using Email for Personal Relationships," *American Behavioral Scientist*, 45, no.3, (November 2001).

Brainerd, Elaine, "School Health Nursing Services Profess Review: Report of 1996 National Meeting," *Journal of School Health*, Vol. 68, No.1, January 1998.

Branham, Chris, "UA addresses need for more male nurses: stereotypes abound," *Arkansas Democratic Gazette*, (July 12, 2004).

182

Brown, Susan and Dorothy Grimes, "Who's number one in primary care, RNs or MDs ?" *RN*, Vol.59, No. 4, April, 1996.

Buerhaus, Peter I., and Douglas O. Staiger, "Future of the Nurse Labor Market According to Executives in High-Managed Care Areas of the United States," *Image: Journal of Nursing Scholarship*, Vol. 29, No. 4, Fourth Quarter, 1997.

Buxman,, Karyn, "Make room for laughter," *American Journal of Nursing*, 91, (December 1991).

Cohen, Albert K. and James F. Short, Jr. , "Research in Delinquent Sub-cultures," *Journal of Social Issues*, 14, (1958).

Cook, Circe, " Reflections on the Health Care Team: My Experiences in an Interdisciplinary Program." *JAMA*, Vol.277, No. 13, April 2, 1997.

Crocker, John and K.M. McGraw, "What's Good for the Goose is not Good for the Gander: Social Status as an Obstacle to Occupational Achievement for Males and Females," *American Behavioral Scientist*, 27, no.3, (1984).

Cromley, Janet, "When Your Doctor is a Nurse," *Good Housekeeping*, " Vol. 225, No.2, August 1997.

Davis-Martin, Shirley, "Research on Males in Nursing," *Journal of Nursing Education*, Vol. 23, No. 4, April 1984.

DeLeon, Patrick H., Diane K. Kjervik, Alan G. Kraut and Gary R. Vanden Bos, "Psychology and Nursing: A Natural Alliance, *American Psychologist*, Vol.40, No. 11, November 1985.

Dentler, Robert A. and Kai T. Erikson, " The Functions of Deviance in Groups," *Social Problems*, 7(Fall 1959).

Dossey, Larry, Space, Time & Medicine, *New Science Library*, Boston, 1982.

Durkheim, Emile, "The Normal and the Pathological," in: Henry N. Potell, editor, *Social Deviance*, (Upper Saddle River, N.J. Pearson, Prentice Hall, 2005).

Dworkin , A.G., J.S. Chafetz and R. Dworkin, "The Effects of Tokenism on Work Alienation," *Work and Occupation*, (August 1986).

Egeland , J., and Julie Brown, "Sex role stereotyping and role strain of male registered nurses." *Research in Nursing and Health*, 11, (1988).

Epstein, Charles, "Encountering the male establishment: Sex-status limits on women's careers in the professions," *American Journal of Sociology*, 75, (1970).

Erikson, Kai T., "Notes on the Sociology of Deviance," *Social Problems*, 9, (1962).

Evans, John, "Men in nursing: issues of gender segregation and hidden advantage" *Journal of Advanced Nursing*, 26 (1997).

Evans, Olga and Andrew Steptoe, "The contribution of gender role orientation, work factors and home stressors to psychological well-being and sickness absence in male and female dominated occupational groups," *Social Science and Medicine*, 54, no. 4 (*Social Science and Medicine*, February 4, 2002.

Falk, Gerhard, *Sex, Gender and Social Change: The Great Revolution*, (New York, University Press of America, 1998).

Falk, Gerhard, *Stigma: How We Treat Outsiders*, (Amherst, N.Y. Prometheus Books, 2001).

Festinger, Leon, *A Theory of Cognitive Dissonance*, (Stanford, Cal. Stanford University Press, 1957).

Fisher, Marshall, "Sex role characteristics of males in nursing." *Contemporary Nurse*, 8, no.3 (1999).

Fisher, Murray, "Stereotypes of male nurses live on," *Nursing Review*, no.3 (March 2002).

Floge, Lilianne and Deborah M. Merrill, "Tokenism Reconsidered: Male Nurses and Female Physicians in a Hospital Setting," *Social Forces*, 64, (1986).

Fottler, Myron D., "Attitudes of Female Nurses Toward the Male Nurse: A Study of Occupational Segregation," *Journal of Health and Social Behavior*, 17, no. 2 (June 1976).

Freudenheim, Milt, "Nurses Treading on Doctor's Turf," *The New York Times*, Nov. 2, 1997.

Galbraith, Michael, "Attracting Men to Nursing: What Will They Find Important in Their Career?" *Journal of Nursing Education*, Vol. 30, No.4, April 1991.

Garfinkel, Harold, "Successful Degradation Ceremonies," *American Journal of Sociology*, 61, (1956).

Gibbs, Jack P. and Maynard J. Erickson, "Major Developments in the Sociological Study of Deviance," *Annual Review of Sociology*, 1, (1975).

Giuffre, Patti A. and Christine L. Williams, "Not Just Bodies: Strategies for Desexualizing the Physical Examination of Patients," *Gender and Society*, 14, no.3, (June 2000).

Gordon, Suzanne, "The Quality of Mercy," *The Atlantic Monthly*, Vol. 279, No. 2, February,1979.

Gutek, Barbara A. and B. Morasch, "Sex-Ratios, Sex-Role Spillover, and Sexual Harassment of Women at Work," *Journal of Social Issues*, 38, no.4, (1982).

Hartman, Heidi, "Capitalism, Patriarchy and Job Segregation by Sex, in: M. Blaxall and B.B. Reagan, Editors. *Women and the Workplace*, (Chicago, University of Chicago Press, 1976).

Helmlinger, Connie, "ANA Hails Landmark Law as Nursing Victory," *AJN* Vol. 97, No. 10, October 1997.

Hess, Beth B., Elizabeth W. Markson and Peter J. Stein, *Sociology*, New York, Macmillan Publishing Co., 1991.

Heymann, Stanley J., "Patients in Research: Not just subjects, but partners." *Science*, Vol. 269.

Hunter, Lauren and Vanda Lops, "Certified Nurse Midwives," *JAMA*, Vol. 277, No.13, April 2, 1997.

Hyman, Herbert, "The Value Systems of Different Classes," in: Reinhard Bendix and Seymour Martin Lipset, Editors, *Class, Status and Power* (New York; The Free Press, 1966).

Joel, Lucille A., "Your License to Practice," *American Journal of Nursing*, Vol.95, No. 11, November 1995.

Johnson, Margie, Susan Goad and Britt Canada, "Attitudes towards Nursing as Expressed by Nursing and Non-nursing College Males," *Journal of Nursing Education*, 3, no.9, (November 1984).

The Journal of Continuing Education in Nursing, Vol.29, No. 1, January/February 1998.

Kalisch, Philip A. and Beatrice Kalisch, *The Advance of American Nursing*, (Philadephia, J.B. Lippincott Co., 1995).

Kalist, David E., "The gender earnings gap in the RN labor market," *Nursing Economics*, 20, no.4, (2002).

Kanter, Rosabeth Moss, Some Effects of Proportions on Group Life: Skewed Sex Ratios and Responses by Token Women," *American Journal of Sociology*, 82, no.5. (1977).

Kaplan, Howard B., Robert J. Johnson and Carol A. Bailey, "Self-rejection and the explanation of deviance," *Social Psychology Quarterly*, 49, no.2, (June 1986).

Keepnews, David, "New Opportunities and Challenges for APRNs." *AJN*, Vol. 98, No.1, January 1998.

Kelly, Carole, "Surveyeing Public Health Nurses' Continuing Education Needs: Collaboration of Practice and Academia," The Journal of Continuing Education in Nursing, Vol. 25, No3, May-June 1997.

Kenyon, Virginia, et al, "Clinical competencies for community health nurses," *Public Health Nursing*, Vol. 7, No. 1, 1990, pp. 33-39.

Kilborn, Peter T., "Nurses Get New Role in Patient Protection," *The New York Times*, March 26, 1998.

Lemert, Edwin M, Human Deviance, *Social Problems and Social Control*, (Englewood Cliffs, N.J., Prentice-Hall, 1967).

Lindberg, Janice B., Mary Love Hunter and Ann Z. Kruszewski, *Introduction to Nursing*, Philadelphia, Lipppincott-Raven Publishers, 1998.

Macionis, John J., *Society: The Basics*, (Upper Saddle River, N.J., Prentice Hall, 2004).

Marx, Gary T., "Ironies of Social Control," *Social Problems*, 28:3 (February 1981).

Merton, Robert K., "Social Structure and Anomie," *American Sociological Review*, 3, (October 1938).

Merton, Robert K., *Social Theory and Social Structure*, New York: The Free Press, (1957).

Meyer, Katherine A., "An Educational Program to Prepare Acute Care Nurses for a Transition to Home Health Care Nursing," *The Journal of Continuing Education in Nursing*, Vol.28, No. 3, May/June 1987.

Moore, Art, "Hospice Care Hijacked," *Christianity Today*, Vol.42, No.3, March 2, 1998.

Muhlenkamp, Albert and John Parsons, "Characteristics of Nurses," *Journal of Vocational Behavior*, 2, (1972).

Nagelkerk, Jean, Patricia M. Ritola and Patty J. Vandort, "Nursing Informatics: The Trend of the Future."

Oppenheimer, Victor, "The sex labeling of jobs," *Industrial Relations*, 7, (1968).

Oransky, Ivan and Jay Varma, "Non-physicians Clinicians and the Future of Medicine," *JAMA*, Vol.277, No. 13, April 2, 1007.

Orlansky, Michael D. and William L. Heward, *Voices: Interviews with Handicapped People* (Columbus, Merrill, 1981).

Orlovsky, Christian, "Survey Says: Nurse Salary on the Rise," *NurseZone.Com* (November 11,2004).

Parsons, Talcott, "Age and Sex in the Social Structure of the United States," in Logan Wilson and William L. Kolb, Editors, *Sociological Analysis*, (New York: Harcourt, Brace and Co. 1949).

Paterson, Barbara L., "The Negotiated Order of Clinical Teaching," *Journal of Nursing Education*, Vol.36, No. 5, May 1997.

Plummer, Kenneth, "Misunderstanding Labeling Perspectives," in David Downes and Paul Rock, Editors, *Deviant Interpretations* (London: Martin Robertson, 1979).

Roberts Joan J., and Thetis M. *Group, Feminism in Nursing* (Westport, Con. Praeger, 1995).

Schultz, Victor, "Reconceptualizing sexual harassment," *Yale Law Journal*, 107, (1998).

Segal, Bernard E., "Male Nurses: A Case Study in Status Contradiction and Prestige Loss," *Social Forces*, 41, no. 1 (October 1962).

Sherman, Deborah Witt, "Correlates of Death Anxiety in Nurses Who Provide AIDS Care," *Omega*, Vol. 34, No.2, 1996-1997.

Sherrod, Roy A, "The Role of the Nurse Educator: When the Obstetrical Nursing Student is Male," *Journal of Nursing Education*, Vol.28, No.8, October 1989.

Sherrod, Roy A., "The Role of the Nurse-Educator when the Obstetrical Nursing Student is Male," *Journal of Nursing Education*, 28, no.8, (October 1989).

Shute, Nancy, "A surge in graduate programs for nurses," *U.S. News and World Report*, March 2, 1998.

Sikoloff, Natalie, *Between Money and Love* (New York: Praeger, 1990).

Sorlie, Venke, Anders Lindseth, Reidun Forde and Astrid Norberg, "The meaning of being in ethically difficult care situations in pediatrics as narrated by male registered nurses," *Journal of Pediatric Nursing*, 18, no.5, (October 2003).

South, Scott J., Charles M. Bonjean, William T. Markham and Judy Corder, "Social Structure and Inter-group Interaction: Men and Women of the Federal Bureaucracy," *American Sociological Review*, 47(1982).

Stamler, Lynette Leeseberg, and Barbara Thomas, "Patient Stories: A Way to Enhance Continuing Education," *Journal of Continuing Education in Nursing*, Vol. 28, No. 2, March/April 1997.

Steubert, Helen J., "Male Nursing Students' Perception of Clinical Experience," *Nurse Educator*, Vol. 19, No.5, September-October 1994.

Stuck, H.E. and H.U.D. Aronow, "A trial of annual in-home comprehensive geriatric assessments for elderly people living in the community," *New England Journal of Medicine*, Vol. 333, No. 18, 1995.

Sutherland, Edwin H., Donald R. Cressey and David F. Luckenbill, *Principles of Criminology*, (Dix Hills, NY, 1992).

Thomas, Sally and Gale Hume, "Delegation Competencies: Beginning Practitioners' Reflections," *Nurse Educator*, Vol. 23, No. 1, January-February 1998.

Trossman, Susan, "Caring Knows No Gender," *The American Journal of Nursing*, 103, no. 5, (May 2003).

"University of Wisconsin nursing school lures more men," *Wisconsin State Journal*, (September 13, 2004).

Vaughan, Jeanette, "Is There Really Racism in Nursing?" *Journal of Nursing Education*, Vol. 36, No. 3, March 1997.

Weber, Max, *The Protestant Ethic and the Spirit of Capitalism*, Talcott Parsons, Trans. (New York: Scribner, 1956.)

Weinberg, Thomas S., *Gay Men, Gay Selves* (New York: Irvington Publishers, 1983).

Williams, Christine L. and E. Joel Heikes, *Gender and Society*, 7, no.2 (June 1993).

Index

A

Acute care specialization, 19
advanced practice registered nurses, 15, 20
advanced technology, 28, 137
AIDS patients, 21
American Association of Colleges of
  Nursing, 17, 26
American Nurses Association, 15, 18
American society, 6, 8, 138, 147
ancillaries, 33
ascribed status, 142-43, 146
assisted suicide, 24

B

Balanced Budget Act, 14-15
Becker, Howard, 1
Bellevue Hospital, 133

C

care situations, 17, 137
chaperones, 152-53
child care, 25, 168
cognitive dissonance, 148-50, 155
Cohen, Albert, 6
Community Nursing Organization, 14
costs of medical care, 13

D

death, 8, 21-23, 44, 48, 63-65, 67-69, 74, 98,
  103-04, 112-13, 131, 159, 163, 177
death anxiety, 21-22
deviance, 1-9, 79, 133, 143, 175
deviant, 1-9, 81-82, 88, 90, 104, 125, 131,
  143, 159-60, 175
difference in communication, 149
differential association, 5-6
dilemma, 64, 148

doctors, 14-15, 18, 20, 22, 26, 29-30, 36-38,
  45, 95, 113, 137-39, 142, 144, 146-48,
  150-51, 153-54, 163, 178
  primary care, 14, 26, 32, 45, 113
dying patient, 22-23

F

Festinger, Leon, 148
Fottler, Myron, 150

G

gender role conflict, 35, 136

H

health care executives, salaries, 29
health care organizations, 16
health care programs, sponsored, 26
health delivery workers, 17
health related professions, 19, 29, 145
Hippocrates, 13
HMOs, 24, 32
home health care, 16-20, 23
homosexuality, 134, 143, 147, 149, 151
hospice, 23, 24
Hospice Foundation of America, 24
hospital(s), 2, 11, 13, 16-18, 20, 23, 27-33,
  37-38, 43, 44, 46, 50-51, 54, 56, 59-60, 63,
  69-70, 72-76, 90, 94, 96-97, 101-02, 107,
  110-14, 116, 125-27, 130, 133, 135, 140,
  144, 146-47, 151, 161-62, 164, 167-69,
  177-78
  cost cutting, 32
  experiences, 23, 27, 31, 34, 48, 84, 167
  legal liability, 28
hospital administrators, 13, 37